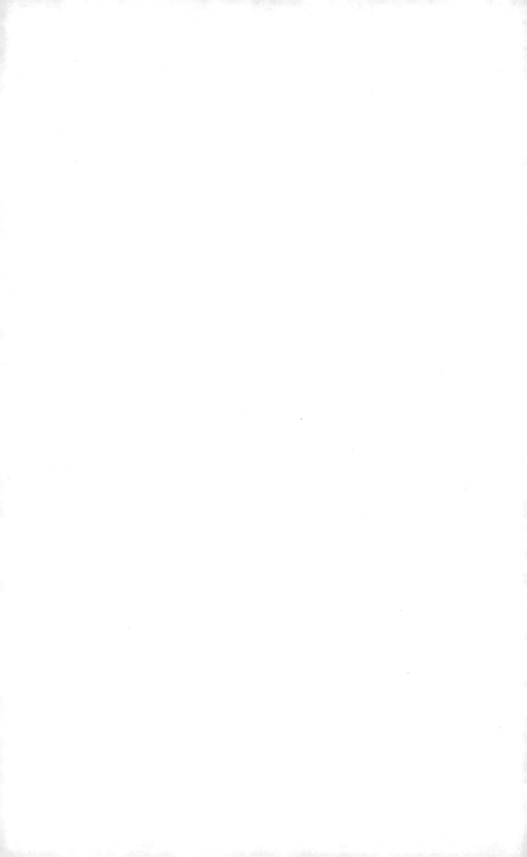

Patient Safety Ethics

Patient Safety Ethics

How Vigilance, Mindfulness, Compliance, and Humility Can Make Healthcare Safer

John D. Banja

 Johns Hopkins University Press   Baltimore

This book was brought to publication through the generous
assistance of the David E. Ryer Director's Endowment.

Johns Hopkins University Press
2715 North Charles Street
Baltimore, Maryland 21218-4363
www.press.jhu.edu

Library of Congress Cataloging-in-Publication Data
Names: Banja, John D., author.
Title: Patient safety ethics : how vigilance, mindfulness, compliance, and humility
    can make healthcare safer / John D. Banja.
Description: Baltimore : Johns Hopkins University Press, 2019 | Includes bibli-
    ographical references and index.
Identifiers: LCCN 2018039681| ISBN 9781421429083 (hardcover : alk. paper) | ISBN
    142142908X (hardcover : alk. paper) | ISBN 9781421429090 (electronic) | ISBN
    1421429098 (electronic)
Subjects: | MESH: Ethics, Clinical | Medical Errors—ethics | Patient Safety | Quality
    of Health Care—ethics
Classification: LCC R729.8 | NLM WB 60 | DDC 610.28/9—dc23
LC record available at https://lccn.loc.gov/2018039681

A catalog record for this book is available from the British Library.

*Special discounts are available for bulk purchases of this book. For more information,
please contact Special Sales at 410-516-6936 or specialsales@press.jhu.edu.*

Johns Hopkins University Press uses environmentally friendly book materials,
including recycled text paper that is composed of at least 30 percent post-
consumer waste, whenever possible.

To my grandchildren:

Emma Lee
Matthew
Michael
Sarah

May they always be reasonably safe

Contents

Preface

The goal of this book is to envision the principles and constitutive elements of patient safety ethics as well as how their related safety practices might be enhanced. Just as Tom Beauchamp and James Childress gave us the principles of autonomy, nonmaleficence, beneficence, and justice as primary conceptual structures illuminating and fueling controversies in bioethics, I propose in this book that vigilance, mindfulness, compliance, and humility are the bedrock of health professionals' ethical obligation to protect their patients from preventable harm.[1]

Consequently, the chapters in this book are devoted to justifying this claim and describing the practical applications of these notions in health-care environments. For illustration, I frequently advert to an informational source not much used in medical ethics, namely, medical malpractice cases. Bioethicists might ignore or dismiss this knowledge source, perhaps thinking that it has little ethical content or value. Unless one has access to the multiple and usually complex stories that plaintiffs and defendants tell in malpractice actions—especially as recorded in depositions—malpractice cases described in the popular press may seem more like sensational examples of appalling carelessness than of ethically fraught situations. Also, the primary goal of medical malpractice suits is commonly understood as securing a monetary award for the plaintiff (which, for the plaintiff, is the goal) rather than securing ethical wisdom. In addition, only about 5 percent of filed claims proceed to trial, so persons sincerely interested in how legal wisdom or the judicial process might embody ethical aspects of patient safety are faced with the difficulty of finding such informational repositories. My goal, then, is to show how certain medical malpractice cases that I've encountered over the years shed considerable light on patient safety ethics. To my knowledge, this book is the only ethics text to date that presents these stories from an ethical vantage point. What, then, might such moral or ethical wisdom amount to and how does it evolve from or speak to patient safety? Beauchamp and Childress have given us the ethical pillars of respecting patients' rights and liberties, refraining from harm, benefiting others, and treating equally and fairly all persons to whom health professionals have a dutiful relationship. We can import straightaway the admonition to refrain from harming others as a foundational construct in patient safety ethics. The idea of health professionals maintaining an unsafe environment for their patients contradicts, at its core, the profession's avowed and public purpose. Exposing healthcare consumers to an unsafe environment would violate the ethos of medical care both formally and practically: The time-honored understanding of healthcare delivery is to cure patients of their ailments or to alleviate their pain and discomfort. An unsafe clinic or hospital would gainsay those very aspirations and be a contradiction to itself, somewhat like *Monty Python*'s cheese shop that doesn't sell any cheese. On a more practical, performative level, health professionals who do not provide care within the safety parameters required by their professions and regulatory agencies are failing to live up to the expectations of their licensure. Thus, even if they fail to cure or alleviate their patients' ailments, healthcare providers are at least required to adhere to safety standards that apply to their performance and to their practice environments.

A somewhat paradoxical aspect of this book is that the medical malpractice case studies give the impression of focusing on grievous errors, mistakes, or unreasonable departures from the standard of care. Yet, healthcare delivery usually works well if not splendidly in an overwhelming number of cases, despite the occurrence of errors. As Erik Hollnagel and his colleagues point out, system operators are generally quite good at getting things right, and that should be the focus of safety scholarship and research.[2] I have more to say about these ideas in chapter 2, but I wish to point out for now only that I am extremely sympathetic to this view and that this book is inspired by it. So, I propose on the one hand that vigilance, mindfulness, compliance, and humility provide important insights into the architecture of getting things right, but on the other hand that medical malpractice cases can greatly illuminate factors that interfere with acceptable outcomes. In other words, to appreciate how system operators keep a fluid, complex, and dynamic care delivery process afloat, we need to understand the pitfalls and traps that can cause the system to go seriously awry. To that end, I believe an analysis of medical malpractice cases will be helpful, especially as that analysis is informed by the four principles of this book.

The essential project of this book is not to discuss the kinds of legal argumentation that occur in medical malpractice courts but to explore the conceptual and performance parameters of patient safety as an ethical achievement. That goal is informed by responding to the justice question of what degree of safety patients are "owed," and therefore what health professionals' duties and obligations are to comply with relevant safety requirements. Consequently, while certain patient safety considerations clearly speak to Beauchamp and Childress's enduring quartet of ethical principles, in certain ways patient safety lies outside the ambit of familiar bioethical problems, such as informed consent, reproduction rights, transplantation dilemmas, end-of-life decisions, and access to healthcare. Perhaps the overriding variable that invites ethical considerations about patient safety is that health professionals and the social and technological environments within which they practice are always "degraded," never optimal.[3] Thus, the question of what level of safety patients are owed is fraught with conceptual, economic, and organizational variables that interdigitate with the imperfections of human nature and thinking, the physical work environment, and the knowledge deficits that penetrate every clinical encounter. The ethics of patient safety is informed by fundamental challenges that will engage us over the scope of this book, such as grappling with the moral problems that derive from working in remarkably complex and hard-to-navigate environments; having to rely on a cognitive skill set that never runs infallibly and often betrays people without their even realizing it; feeling an intense need to accommodate production quotas and pressures such that professionals will often deviate from rules and standards; and failing to have the moral will to admit one's fallibilities and the imperfections of the work environment interface.

Part I offers an overview of patient safety from the standpoint of ethical theory, followed by a chapter each on the text's four foundational components. So, chapter 1 begins with a brief history of the patient safety movement and then inquires into how patient safety would be understood according to three familiar ethical theories: deontology, utilitarianism, and virtue theory. I then show how the four primary ethical constructs that I'm proposing for patient safety—vigilance, mindfulness, compliance, and humility—would in part address but also distinguish themselves from Beauchamp and Childress's principles of autonomy, nonmaleficence, beneficence, and justice.

Chapter 2, which is divided into two parts, characterizes the concept of vigilance as monitoring the external work environment. In the first part, I offer a conceptual overview of vigilance, foreseeability, and their roles in developing the skill set of what I refer to as a "reasonably cautious person." The second part focuses on the nature of harm: How is harm conceptualized from an ethical perspective? And given the omnipresence and ineradicability of risk, what criteria might determine whether a particular environment's risk exposure is ethically "acceptable"?

In chapter 3, I discuss the idea of mindfulness in the sense of monitoring one's internal mental environment. Mindfulness is represented here not as it exists in Eastern contemplative practices but rather as a way for health professionals to regulate their cognitive performance in safety-enhancing ways.

Compliance, the focus of chapter 4, is often (mis)understood simply as a legal and regulatory burden. But the concept should be appreciated for not only its moral foundations but also the extraordinary frequency with which health professionals violate their organizations' rules, regulations, standards, policies, and procedures. As in the previous chapters on vigilance and mindfulness, in this chapter, I offer some recommendations for achieving a relevant skill set.

Chapter 5 centers on a much-endorsed but little-analyzed concept in the world of harm-causing medical errors: humility. Here I offer a historical and philosophical overview of the topic and examine some anecdotal observations on humility in the practice of medicine—anecdotal because little empirical research is at hand. Nevertheless, considerable empirical and conceptual literature covers *overconfidence* in medicine and how it might contribute to patient harm, especially in the arena of diagnostic error. In this chapter, I also explore whether humility can be taught and how it might be learned.

Part II begins with chapter 6, which takes up several issues raised in chapter 2. In a more theoretical way, I return to the question of how much vigilance healthcare professionals owe to one another and to their patients. I largely argue that theory and philosophical speculation are unavailable to answer this question because the risk of harm is so densely contextualized. We rather frame our ethical obligations on calibrating levels of vigilance according to the peculiarities of the risk environment, along with economic and epistemic contingencies that can vary that obligation as the risk environment itself changes (e.g., through technological, architectural, staffing, and individual preference changes).

Chapter 7 reviews the nature of error and its all-too-numerous manifestations; its acknowledgment and disclosure; the animus toward error commission, perhaps originating in perfectionist fantasies; and incident reporting. I examine safety from the perspective of its wrongful loss, namely when health professionals are accused in court of harm-causing negligence.

How the medical malpractice framework can be understood as an ethical construct is the focus of chapter 8, with particular focus on the ethical bases of the plaintiff's burden of proof and the interlocking notions of negligence and standard of care. I lament that the courts do relatively little to support health professionals in illuminating the standard of care, largely because few medical malpractice cases wind up going to a jury trial, and fewer still are appealed.

Chapter 9 ends the book by looking toward the near future. The past two decades of the patient safety movement have indeed witnessed some progress, but not to the degree that was anticipated at the turn of this century. The human brain may simply be unable to navigate the challenges imposed by contemporary technological innovation and the production pressures that accompany it. The next two decades, however, may live up to the promise of unprecedented improvement in patient safety, largely through increasingly sophisticated technological systems, especially as they incorporate artificial intelligence.

I was very gratified when a number of experts agreed to be interviewed for this project. I heartily thank Richard Cook, Pat Croskerry, June Price Tangney, Fran Charney, Tommy Malone, and Bob Wachter for their time and wisdom.

And that allows me to segue into a general expression of thanks to those closest to me who have supported my work and helped make my life meaningful. My heartfelt gratitude goes first and foremost to Judy, my wonderful wife of 47 years, who has suffered my narcissism and numerous other faults and foibles with considerable patience, and to the two children she gave me, Mike and Chris, who taught me more about life than any philosophy book ever could. They, in turn, have families, and I am delighted to be called Grampy by four utterly precious grandchildren, to whom I've dedicated this book. And my thanks would be incomplete if I omitted mention of the indescribable joy I have had working at Emory University since 1983. Thanks especially to Paul Root Wolpe, director of the Center for Ethics, and Kathy Kinlaw, associate director, who provided immense moral and material support to me over the years, without which whatever success I've had would have been impossible. I know that one of the most poignant moments of my life will be when I leave the Emory campus for the last time.

On a more pleasant note, my fervent hope is that this book will contribute in some way to making patients safer. In understanding the ethical underpinnings of patient safety, perhaps more health professionals will actively foster changes to substantially reduce the risk of harm among themselves and the human beings they serve. Unfortunately, the effort and learning curve in improving patient safety are never ending, because knowledge, economics, personnel, and technology change unceasingly. But patient safety work is also undeniably as noble as it is important. As long as humans and their technologies remain fallible and imperfect, concerns over patient safety should and will endure.

Patient Safety Ethics

I Patient Safety and Ethical Theory: The Significance of Vigilance, Mindfulness, Compliance, and Humility

1   Ethical Foundations of Patient Safety

> [T]he odds against error-free performance seem overwhelmingly high.
>
> James Reason[1(p2)]

Chapter Overview: This chapter begins with a brief history of the patient safety movement and then situates patient safety ethics within a trio of familiar ethical theories, namely deontology, utilitarianism, and virtue theory. I then compare patient safety obligations and constructs with those familiar from bioethics textbooks, particularly the famous quartet of principles offered by Tom Beauchamp and James Childress in 1979, in their first edition of *Principles of Biomedical Ethics.* Whereas bioethics seems largely concerned with conceptual dilemmas over individual rights, the nature of harm and welfare, and issues bearing on justice and fairness, patient safety ethics primarily targets a single objective: to mitigate risk as much as possible by evolving a skill set informed by hazard awareness. The contents of that skill set include the practices of vigilance, mindfulness, compliance, and humility—the cornerstones of patient safety ethics.

In *Principles of Biomedical Ethics,* Tom Beauchamp and James Childress presented the principles of autonomy, nonmaleficence, beneficence, and justice as foundational to Western bioethical analysis.[2] I am proposing that vigilance, mindfulness, compliance, and humility are similarly constitutive of health professionals' ethical obligation to protect their patients from preventable harm—in effect, that these latter four constructs are to patient safety ethics what Beauchamp and Childress's principles are to traditional bioethical analysis. This book's investigative journey oscillates between the healthcare work environment and the psychomotor performance of its personnel. This approach invites an appreciation of health professionals' anxieties and epistemic challenges, brought on by caring for very ill and sometimes extremely demanding patients (and families), as well as by working in remarkably complex systems, with processes ranging from thoroughly unstandardized (with little performance reliability or consistency from person to person) to systems tightly regulated by complex policies, procedures, rules, regulations, and standards.

The fundamental challenge of patient safety is that all human, material, and operational components of the healthcare system are imperfect—from the personnel, whose knowledge bases are incomplete, whose memories are fallible, and whose decisional and perceptual skills are vulnerable, to the messy environments in which they work, where other people, complex technologies, and countless processes that occur second by second never function perfectly yet usually deliver a reasonably good product. Indeed, the latter observation demands our attention: If system operators are so vulnerable to error, and if they work in environments where error traps and pitfalls abound, how is it that personnel usually perform admirably or at least without significant mishap?

These challenges to and questions about patient safety need a conceptual underpinning that goes some way to explaining how patient safety is a fundamentally ethical project. A natural urge is to jump directly into improvement processes without first appreciating the more implicit notions that undergird safety obligations—in addition to, of course, the glaringly obvious "above all, do no harm" injunction that has come down to us from the Hippocratic tradition.[3]

Consequently, I begin with a brief history of how, over the past 30 years, patient safety has come to be regarded as a matter of immense professional concern, and then discuss how patient safety might be ethically represented or framed, at least according to three familiar ethical paradigms: deontology, utilitarianism, and virtue theory. The chapter ends with some ethical context on the four themes that will engage us for the remainder of the book: vigilance, mindfulness, compliance, and humility. Most of these analyses use illustrative materials from medical malpractice cases I've consulted on over the years. The goal is to show how such cases offer important insights into how things can go wrong in healthcare, the extent to which we can hold health professionals accountable when processes go awry and outcomes are suboptimal, and the kinds of obligations and practices we can reasonably impose on personnel providing healthcare in early twenty-first-century environments.

Some History on the Patient Safety Movement

During the twentieth century, anesthesiologists were probably the medical specialty group most interested and active in enhancing patient safety.

Perhaps acutely embarrassed by an ABC special on *20/20* in 1982 that focused on anesthesia errors resulting in injuries or death, the American Society of Anesthesiologists created the Anesthesia Patient Safety Foundation (APSF) in 1985.[4,5] As a result, certain anesthesia practices, like pulse oximetry and electronic monitoring, became standardized, and in just a few years, the anesthesia-related death rate plummeted from about 2 in 10,000 to 1 in 200,000–300,000.[6]

Nevertheless, and despite some noteworthy events that should have galvanized public attention to medical errors, the twentieth century was not notable for fostering a practical or intentional approach to patient safety, perhaps because the topic was humiliating and anxiety provoking for physicians and hospital organizations. Also, for most of the century, healthcare consumers tended to be docile and passive, such that most would not seriously pursue the idea of malpractice litigation, even if they suspected something had gone terribly awry, causing injury to themselves or to loved ones.[7] During my adolescence in the 1960s, two of my uncles died in hospitals under mysterious circumstances, and an aunt was discharged from the hospital with an obvious and permanent cognitive impairment that most likely was caused by a hypoxic or anoxic event. No explanations were ever forthcoming, and my relatives were too shy to ask.

This reluctance to hold the healthcare delivery industry more accountable is remarkable given some of the historical events that should have triggered a patient safety movement during the last decades of the twentieth century. Lucian Leape, a founder of the safety movement, recalled several such examples in a 2008 essay:

- The Harvard Medical Practice Study, which appeared in the *New England Journal of Medicine* in 1991, reported that 3.7 percent of hospitalized patients in acute care hospitals in New York State in 1984 experienced iatrogenic harm; 69 percent of those incidents were caused by error and so were preventable; 14 percent of the total were fatal.
- "[A] pivotal year for patient safety" was 1995, with wrong-side surgeries in the news along with the nationally reported case of Betsy Lehman, a *Boston Globe* health reporter who received massive, ultimately lethal doses of chemotherapy by mistake.[8(p4)]
- In 1996 the first multidisciplinary conference on medical errors was held at the Annenberg Center for Health Sciences in California, where the American Medical Association (AMA) announced the formation of

the National Patient Safety Foundation; Diane Vaughan introduced her theory of the "normalization of deviance," which I chronicle in chapter 4; and Ben Kolb's tragic death from medication error was described as a case study in error disclosure with full transparency (also discussed in the Richard Cook interview in chapter 2).

- From 1996 until November 1999, multiple patient safety initiatives began to form, including computerized physician-order entry, bar codes to prevent medication errors, pharmacist participation in intensive care rounds, and simulation training in hospitals and in healthcare educational curricula.[8]

Yet, as Leape noted, "patient safety was not a major concern for most hospitals or doctors, nor for the public, until November of 1999 when the IOM [Institute of Medicine] released its report *To Err Is Human*."[8(p4)] On the first page of that paper was the attention-grabbing statement that would be quoted on just about every evening news program the day the report was released: "[A]t least 44,000 Americans die each year as a result of medical errors . . . and the number may be as high as 98,000."[6(p1)] An astute *New York Times Magazine* journalist, Michael M. Weinstein, noted that if those numbers were correct, then the yearly death rates from medical errors were equivalent to the rates expected if three jumbo jets crashed every two days: "If the airlines killed that many people annually," Weinstein observed, "public outrage would close them overnight."[9]

Analogizing medical errors to air fatalities grabbed the moral conscience of US political leadership. Congress acted rapidly, appropriating $50 million to the Agency for Healthcare Research and Quality to distribute as grants to organizations for research and interventions intended to improve patient safety.[10] The Georgia Hospital Association (GHA) successfully applied for an award, and in a remarkable stroke of good fortune, I was asked to participate on the GHA project; since that time, I have devoted a substantial portion of my professional life to studying medical errors and their appearance in medical malpractice actions.

One of my first projects on the GHA grant in 2002, to develop an instructional video on disclosing medical errors, illustrates how attitudes toward patient safety were in transition back then. As a medical ethicist, I simply took it for granted that if a serious, harm-causing error occurred, then the involved health professionals would disclose that error to the injured parties in a reasonably clear, truthful, and comprehensive way. I developed a video script embodying those premises and presented it to the GHA leadership, who were largely fine with it. The problem arose when a group of defense lawyers from around the state, who advised the GHA on legal matters, saw the script and were flabbergasted over the disclosure proposal. Up until then, it had been customary to conceal such information from harmed parties to avoid compromising the liability of the health professional or the hospital.[11(pp19–46)] In law, this concealment of an "admission against interest" is justified and persists today, such as in automobile insurance policies that discourage policyholders from admitting liability, which can include saying, "I'm sorry."[12] Some of the lawyers in the group even strong-armed the GHA by saying that if the association produced and distributed the video, they would urge their clients in hospital leadership and personnel not to watch it. Fortunately, peace prevailed when we hit on the idea of devoting the first half of the video to a panel discussion featuring two hospital lawyers and a risk manager. Each had an opportunity to offer his or her insights, which largely corroborated my initial belief that harm-causing error should be disclosed. (Unfortunately, the video is no longer available.) Today, not even 20 years later, I think it safe to say that few people would publicly endorse that lawyer group's recommendation as ethical. Concealing a serious harm-causing error from an injured party would seem morally revolting and ethically indefensible. Furthermore, if such a case went to court, the plaintiff's lawyer would relish the opportunity to characterize such a concealment as an example of the defendants' unscrupulousness.

I discussed this kind of situation in my 2005 book, *Medical Errors and Medical Narcissism*, arguing that such concealment violated an ethic of patient centeredness.[11] Today, the ethical formation of patient safety has, I believe, shifted to something like the following: Healthcare consumers in the twenty-first century have become much more informed, suspicious, and aggressive about the behaviors and practices of health professionals, owing in part to the managed care revolution of the last 30 years. For example, and in stark contrast to the era I remember from the 1960s and '70s, a familiar refrain in contemporary risk management is that error concealment will increase the probability of a lawsuit and its cost.[13] The reason is that patients and families often suspect that something has gone wrong, and the stonewalling health professional will likely provoke their suspicion and anger, perhaps prompting a lawsuit. Much of the twenty-first-century thrust on patient safety, which continues the inspiration of *To Err Is Human*, is no longer to conceal error occurrences but to study their conditions and take aggressive, affirmative steps to reduce their frequency and severity.[14]

And that is the tack this book takes. I am interested in placing that etiology of errors and lapses in patient safety in an ethical context. In what follows, I establish patient safety as a bona fide ethical topic by situating it within three familiar ethical frameworks: deontology, utilitarianism, and virtue. Readers who are disinterested in this more philosophical treatment might skip ahead to "Classical Bioethics and Patient Safety Ethics," where the discussion becomes more contextualized and practical. There I offer a glimpse of subsequent chapters, in which I discuss what I take to be quintessential skills and sensibilities required for twenty-first-century patient safety ethics.

Situating Patient Safety within Ethical Theory

Because this book is intended for an audience of in-the-trenches healthcare providers and their leaders rather than professional philosophers, some admittedly light but nevertheless important consideration should be given to how time-honored ethical theories like deontology, utilitarianism, and virtue theory underpin our patient safety sensibilities. In the following sections, I briefly make those observations and illustrate certain points with case examples from medical malpractice as well as a Florida patient safety event that garnered public attention.

Deontological Aspects of Patient Safety

How might a *deontologist* understand patient safety? Such a person is concerned about what duty requires (*deontos* is the Greek word for duty), and the requirements of duty are admittedly shaped by cultures.[15] Still, and even though most duties are cultural inventions and therefore can differ dramatically from group to group, we should remind ourselves that healthcare professionals formally hold themselves out to the public as capable practitioners, especially through their licenses and certifications. Health professionals make an explicit promise to the public not to harm intentionally but to be reasonably compliant with care practices that seek the patient's benefit.[16] Obviously, if consumers of professional services should be able to assume anything as they consider receiving care from licensed or certified professionals, it is that they will not be unnecessarily or unreasonably harmed. Thus, when a client or patient does suffer *unnecessary or reasonably preventable* harm, the professional has failed to uphold his or her dutiful promise of delivering competent, standard-of-care services. In effect, the professional has failed to exercise reasonable caution and skill as anticipated by whatever professional standard-of-care policy applies.[17]

The eighteenth-century philosopher Immanuel Kant famously bequeathed the "categorical imperative" to the West, which represents his attempt to articulate ethical principles according to the "universality" of reason, or reflecting his notion of the "moral law."[18] The imperative—act so that the maxim of your act can become a universal law—is usually interpreted to mean that if we can imagine an action and its supporting rationale or justification played out over a "universe" of cases, then morally appropriate behavior will be tokened by the action's rational consistency or non-contradictoriness *over that universe of cases.* In other words, the practice and its supporting rationale will not prove self-defeating but will survive all its instantiations or imaginings as logically consistent.[19] Applying that reasoning to healthcare, health professionals who promise not to harm unnecessarily but who then do exactly that through error or carelessness—think of wrong site or wrong patient surgeries, catastrophic medication errors, or lost mammograms or lab tests that result in unjustifiable and harmful treatment delays—have contradicted their professional promise to the public. Even though the failure is likely not intentional, as an error, it was preventable. One cannot both claim to practice according to an ethical code informed by professional standards and then commit harm through fault, that is, through negligence or carelessness.[6,13,20] This is why error will often translate into a keen source of psychological distress for clinicians, because erring professionals must deal with the cognitive dissonance between presenting a public image as competent healers and then failing to accommodate that image.[21] The error also introduces the psychological impact of Kant's notion of self-contradiction: it is hard to be emotionally well when you steadfastly promise one good thing but sometimes do a bad thing and then try to conceal it.

Notice, too, how a *contractualist* theory supplements the deontological sensibility in grounding the duty of health professionals in their promissory actions. They take professional oaths; hospitals make glowing, public promises to potential consumers on highway billboards; and medical training programs boast about the caliber of their students, their pass rates on licensing examinations, and the quality of their learning experiences. While health professionals' performance is usually acceptable, committing a serious harm-causing error can be extremely painful, and professionals sometimes understandably resort to psychological mechanisms like denial, rationalization, or minimization of what happened to relieve themselves of the anguish.[11] In more extreme cases, some professionals have left health-care, and a few have taken their own lives.[22]

A duty-based ethic therefore offers a ready theoretical construct for comprehending patient safety as an ethical obligation anchored in the consistency of professionals' dutiful accommodation of their clients' fundamental right not to be harmed by any reasonably preventable event. A problem with this framework, however, is that it begs the question of the *extent* of professionals' duty to ensure patient safety. Duties are not only shaped by social expectations but constrained by the practical realities of the environment. Health professionals' performance can be influenced by the quality of technology they use, the level of training and skill they possess, and the production demands that confront them, such as the number of patients to see, the technological and human resources at their disposal, and so forth.[23] Consider how these variables complicate determining the extent of the healthcare provider's duty to patient safety in the following cases:

Case 1.1. A patient with an allergy to sulfa drugs was admitted to the hospital. Although she informed multiple caretakers of her drug allergy, that information was never transferred to the *allergy drop-down box* of her electronic medical record. Other parts of her record documented her allergy, however, such as her medical history notes and a consultation report. On the morning of her discharge, her lab reports indicated that she was developing an infection, and her attending physician ordered Bactrim, a sulfa-based antibiotic to which she was allergic. Ninety minutes later, she began showing classic signs of an allergic reaction, and two days later, she was dead. The physician was sued but pleaded that he had fulfilled his professional duties by examining the allergy drop-down box, which he had. In effect, he argued that he had "inherited" an error—the failure to note the patient's drug allergy appropriately—that was not his fault. When he didn't see the allergy listed, he believed that searching other parts of the patient's records to gather additional drug information was unnecessary, that is, not required by his standard-of-care obligations.

Case 1.2. A nurse received an order to set up an infusion pump that delivers a one-liter bag of medicine to a patient who has unintentionally taken a drug overdose. The drug delivery protocol was complex, requiring varying flow rates over a 21-hour period, and the nurse had never delivered the medicine before. She programmed the infusion delivery rate *exactly as the physician's order dictated*, but the physician's order contained a 16-fold overdose error, which was not discovered until nearly two days later, during which time the patient had received the medicine more or less continuously. The patient was discharged to another facility but within hours deteriorated to a vegetative state. At the nurse's deposition, she denied allegations that she should have been aware of the dosage error by checking the order against a formulary or some authoritative source before administering the medicine. She claimed that a nurse should be able to depend on the accuracy of a physician's order and that her dutiful obligations required only that she deliver the medication exactly as written on the order.

Each of these examples illustrates the problems a duty-oriented approach would encounter in deciding the moral propriety of the actors. Were the clinicians' arguments—that they sufficiently dispatched their duties despite the resulting harm—acceptable or not? We return to these cases in subsequent chapters, but for now, we can examine whether deontology's great competitor theory, utilitarianism, might better address the ethical questions that arise in the context of patient safety.

Improving Welfare: The Utilitarian Perspective

One of the ethical themes that reverberates throughout this book is how the idea of a reasonably cautious person plays a central role in patient safety practices and policy formation. The intent of such cautiousness is obviously patient centered because patients (as well as personnel) are the rightful beneficiaries of safety efforts and attitudes.[23] Indeed, the exercise of reasonable caution in healthcare delivery is quintessential to why things go right so often. The argument is not that reasonably cautious persons are errorless, but that they are continuously monitoring the environment for harm opportunities and aggressively taking corrective action when they spot them.

Nonetheless, aspiring toward ever greater levels of patient safety also has "costs." Indeed, and reminiscent of drug discovery in the twentieth century, the more a healthcare organization and personnel drill down into the deeper strata of patient safety practices, policies, and technological and economic infrastructures, the more costly the safety enterprise becomes. Because pharmacologic discovery may well have picked much of the "low-hanging fruit" in the latter half of the twentieth century, drug research today is much more expensive because its experiments require more exotic, expensive science and supportive technologies.[25] Just so, achieving ever greater levels of patient safety requires increasing investment in goof-proof technologies, better-trained staff, and a more comprehensive system of tracking errors that feeds the lessons learned back into the system.[26]

Utilitarians are sensitive to these cost-benefit trade-offs because they recognize that outcomes or consequences are morally evaluated according to the preferences of some group.[27] And while different groups may have different preferences, economic constraints undeniably affect the possibilities that contemporary professionals can offer patients and, by extension, the scope of what exercising "reasonable caution" entails in such circumstances. Thus, the hospital that enjoys excellent economic resources might be able to provide a consistently safer environment and better clinical outcomes than one that is struggling to survive and has to manage with older technologies, a staff whose numbers are cut to the bone, and a continuing medical education budget that rarely allows clinicians any time from routine patient care to attend a training seminar. While the latter situations may seem unacceptable, a utilitarian might nevertheless argue that such a hospital can still accomplish much more good than harm, despite the occasional harm-causing error or a higher percentage of suboptimal outcomes compared to other facilities. Although I do not pursue the argument here, some healthcare institutions have no choice but to expose their patients to higher levels of risk or a likelihood of poorer outcomes because of various contingencies, such as the hospital's inability to consistently attract and maintain a well-trained staff of clinicians.

Some particularly ornery ethical problems reside in this universe of socioeconomic, demographic, resource-capacity, and revenue-generating variables. Consider the 2015 case involving St. Mary's Medical Center in West Palm Beach, Florida. CNN reporters Elizabeth Cohen and John Bonifield painted a troubling picture of the surgical death risk in the hospital's pediatric congenital cardiac surgery program, claiming that the mortality rate for open heart surgeries on children and babies was 12.5 percent from 2011 to 2013, while the national average was 3.3 percent, as cited by the Society for Thoracic Surgeons.[28] While CNN's reporters did not make any allegations of medical malpractice, they noted that according to a report from the Cardiac Technical Advisory Panel of expert pediatric cardiologists, St. Mary's was not doing a *sufficient number* of pediatric cardiac procedures to gain adequate expertise in managing the risks and treatment challenges inherent in these complex surgeries. The panel also believed that the hospital had inadequate echocardiogram reports and insufficient pediatric electrophysiology expertise and resources. At least 6 babies died during the two-year interval of 48 cases—thus CNN's mortality rate estimation of 12.5 percent—prompting the panel to advise that the program not perform further surgeries until its alleged deficiencies were remediated.[28]

Most of the children who died at St. Mary's were reported to be on Medicaid, which, despite its reputation as a poor source of reimbursement, in fact paid Florida's hospitals extremely well for these pediatric cardiac surgeries.[29] The CNN reports thus appeared to suggest that if St. Mary's was sufficiently aware of its poor outcomes but performed the surgeries anyway, then Medicaid's generous reimbursement may have played more than a minor (and, hence, ethically problematic) role in encouraging the surgical program.

St. Mary's response to these allegations was to repudiate CNN's 12.5 percent mortality rate as "wrong," "exaggerated," and "completely erroneous."[30] The hospital claimed that CNN had used faulty analytics: had the networks' analysts used adequate "risk-adjustment" measures, accounting for factors like the acuity of the pediatric surgical patients who were admitted and the difficulty of the surgery, as well as factoring in closed cardiac procedures in addition to open ones, then the hospital's mortality rate would had reduced to an acceptable 5.3 percent (with the State of Florida claiming that St. Mary's risk-adjusted rate was actually 4.58 percent).[31] St. Mary's did not disclose what risk-adjusted measures it used to arrive at its lower figure, however, so the hospital's claim couldn't be substantiated. Subsequently, St. Mary's closed its pediatric cardiac surgery program in August 2015, claiming that CNN's adverse publicity made it impossible for the program to continue. The chief of the program also filed a defamation suit against the network.[29,32]

This case easily lends itself to a utilitarian analysis focusing on consequences and preferences. If CNN was correct in its charges and claims, the news network probably felt a public health triumph when St. Mary's cardiac program closed down. But if St. Mary's was right that CNN had miscalculated the mortality rate such that the actual rate was in an acceptable range, then the news organization was responsible for the closing of an otherwise valuable program of pediatric health services. Furthermore, CNN's multiple stories must have caused acute anguish in many persons with a stake in St. Mary's success, as well as in the families who came to the conclusion that their children were unnecessarily harmed. If CNN's stories were ultimately false or baseless, then they had caused numerous harms without any offsetting benefits, which would make utilitarians cringe.

The utilitarian argument for patient safety is obvious: People will not access healthcare if doing so results in their being worse off. So they will, all other things being equal, gravitate to care providers who offer comparatively safer and better care. This CNN story illustrates how high the stakes are in patient safety, how emotions will run equally high because human welfare and professional careers are also at stake, and how the involved parties will seek to defend themselves, their interests, and the quality of their work. These phenomena appear time and again in the pages that follow because they illustrate an important facet of patient safety ethics: because the truth can be elusive, the best way to resolve problems is with logical reasoning, facts that are supported by the best data, and a commitment to transparency, honesty, and good will.

The "Virtuous" Health Professional

In addition to deontological and consequentialist ethical theories, the *virtue ethics* literature dating back to Aristotle suggests a set of habits or dispositions that speaks to patient safety. As Aristotle suggested in *Nicomachean Ethics*, the virtuous person will do the right thing, for the right reason, supported by the right feelings.[33] Virtue ethics typically places a great deal of emphasis on experience or acquired wisdom, which qualifies it as a helpful explanatory construct for thinking about patient safety and avoiding preventable mishaps. While this is especially the case when novel or innovative work factors are introduced, it applies just as well to ordinary and familiar work settings. Here is an example:

Case 1.3. A mother with a long history of drug addiction, including heroin and cocaine abuse, and with numerous admissions to rehab became pregnant and delivered a healthy term baby while she was enrolled in a methadone program. The baby developed neonatal abstinence syndrome and required pharmacologic withdrawal. The drug of choice is morphine given orally. The baby was on a small dose of 0.09 mg every 4 hours. A 10-fold overdose was sent from the pharmacy and administered. Fortunately, this mistake with oral morphine was not dangerous. The oral dose range for *pain control* in the neonate is from 0.15 mg to 1.00 mg/kg per dose every 4 hours. So, for this 3.00 kg baby, an oral pain-control dose range would have been 0.45 to 3.00 mg. The erring dose of 0.90 mg therefore posed no threat to the infant. Should the parents nevertheless be informed about the error?

I still recall the pained look on the physician's face as he recounted this story to me, even though it is a classic example of a "harmless hit," where the medicine reached the patient but no adversity occurred. Thus, a "no harm/no foul" utilitarian-like maxim might justify concealment, but this physician invoked a virtue ethic approach when he disclosed the error to the mother, not just because he felt she had a right to know, but because of the physician's sense of integrity, as when he said, "If I conceal what happened in this case, what's to stop me from concealing in another case and another one—because you can always find a reason not to disclose the truth."

What speaks to the virtuous professional who subscribes to an ethics of disclosure, however, can be generalized to all patient safety. If health professionals are keen to practice in and maintain reasonably safe environments, then that very attitude and its related behaviors must count as virtuous and laudable. When things go wrong, however, we are left with the ethical problem of calculating the degree to which the involved professionals should be held responsible for those wrongs and possibly penalized. Such discernments are sometimes not easy to make because they are highly contextualized; they often elicit emotional reactions from others without good logical justification; and unless good risk-management analysis and response are forthcoming, the actual causes of an adversity might remain unchanged regardless of whichever penalties are imposed on the personnel involved.

Classical Bioethics and Patient Safety Ethics

To gain insight into how bioethics and patient safety ethics can differ, comparing two cases might be helpful. The first is a typical bioethics case coming to a hospital ethics committee, whereas the second introduces the organizing themes of the chapters that follow.

Case 1.4. Mr. Jones was a 32-year-old electrician who became unconscious at work. He was taken by ambulance to a local hospital, admitted to intensive care, and then sent directly to radiology for brain scans. His mother and his bride-to-be arrived at the hospital and were given the worst possible news. Mr. Jones had just been declared brain dead but was being maintained on a respirator so that they could express their farewells. Mr. Jones and his fiancée had planned to be married in five days. After Mrs. Jones and the fiancée recovered their emotional equilibrium, they approached the healthcare team with a request: They asked for Mr. Jones's sperm with the hope that his fiancée could be impregnated and have his offspring. Retrieving the sperm would require an orchiectomy. The hospital had never been confronted with such a request and convened an ethics committee meeting to develop a response.

Case 1.5. Mrs. Smith was a 60-year-old woman who was relatively healthy but needed to have her gall bladder removed. Her laparoscopic cholecystectomy began shortly after noon. All was going well until the surgeon decided that he wanted a cholangiogram, that is, a radiologic image of the area he had been operating on. To do this, an x-ray machine was wheeled over to the side of the patient's bed, the bed was elevated, and the anesthesiologist turned off the ventilator for a few seconds, or just long enough for the image to be taken. When someone tried to lower the bed after the image had been taken, the crank stuck, and the bed remained in the elevated position. When someone else tried to remove the cassette from the x-ray machine to inspect the image, it got stuck in the machine. The anesthesiologist saw what was happening and left his station to help lower the bed and remove the cassette. He failed to turn the ventilator back on, resulting in the patient's going without ventilation for an undetermined length of time. It could have been as long as 20 minutes, but the anesthesiologist did not chart the incident nor the length of time the patient had been without artificial ventilation. No one in the operating room noticed that the patient was "off the vent." When the anesthesiologist discovered his error and turned the ventilator back on, he told no one and hoped the patient would be all right. Tragically, the patient was ultimately left in a vegetative state after her bout of anoxia and spent the next nine days in intensive care, whereupon her family members ultimately consented to her removal from the ventilator. She died two days later. The family was never told about the ventilator error but somehow found out about it and proceeded to sue. A key finding in their negligence suit was that prior to the surgery, a technician had intentionally disabled all the alarms in the operating room at the behest of the hospital's clinical leadership, who complained about the annoyance and irritation the technology caused (a.k.a. "alarm fatigue"). It was also surmised that the anesthesiologist had turned the pulse oximeter down to inaudible. Thus, this disaster was presumably enabled by disabling the very technology that was supposed to prevent it. The case ultimately settled out of court.

Case 1.4 is the kind of scenario with which bioethicists are very familiar. Indeed, we can briefly analyze some of its central issues according to the Beauchamp-Childress *principlist* model.[2]

Autonomy: Whose rights, liberties, freedoms, and choices should prevail in this case? Do the health providers have the right to deny the family's sperm request if they feel uncomfortable about it, or do patients' rights morally require the professionals to overcome their discomfort and accommodate it? Are Mrs. Jones and the fiancée making a rational request, or might their thinking be disturbed by this tragedy such that they will come to regret their request if it is accommodated? Although Mr. Jones is deceased, does he have any rights authority in this situation? Ought we honor his values and wishes even though he will not be able to realize or witness them in any way? How would we know with any degree of confidence what his values might be?

Nonmaleficence: How does "harm" play out in this case? When confronted with the request, some members of the healthcare team balked because the preferred intervention for securing the sperm was an orchiectomy, which some thought was tantamount to "physical mutilation." If the sperm is used and a child is born, would his or her quality of life be acceptable without a father? As time goes on, might the fiancée come to change her mind about this whole arrangement but nevertheless feel coerced to comply with the original plan because of Mr. Jones's sperm residing in some sperm bank? Perhaps she will fall in love again and want to marry, which the presence of Mr. Jones's sperm or children might discourage.

Beneficence: Health professionals work to alleviate physical and emotional suffering. Although they have every right to use their moral values in calculating benefits and goodness in this case, they should not "unreasonably" impose their morality on Mrs. Jones and the fiancée. Consequently, the healthcare team must exercise ethical sensitivity in honoring Mrs. Jones's and the fiancée's autonomy and their right to their own values and comprehension about benefits. At the moment, both women's values are asserting the benefit of having Mr. Jones's offspring, which creates a strong presumptive, or prima facie, claim on having that wish honored.

Justice: The health team must also try to ensure fairness and objectivity in making its decision, and of course, whatever team members decide must accommodate the law. How does the authority to make the final determination play out in this case? How far does either party's right to insist on their preferences extend? What decisional process or methodology should the ethics committee recommend that would embody "fairness" to all concerned?

Ultimately, because Mr. Jones might not want to bring a child into the world that he could not raise and love, and because there was no evidence that Mr. Jones would want a child brought into the world to whom he could never respond as a father, the ethics committee decided that it would be disrespectful to his autonomy—or at least ethically presumptuous—to proceed with the surgery. Mrs. Jones and the fiancée accepted this decision. The point is that this analysis of Case 1.4 raises questions and concerns that are familiar to ethics committees and uses a principlist approach in framing the ethical character of this story.[2] Patient safety ethics presents us with a different set of considerations; yet they are no less professional or moral. So consider the issues pertinent to Case 1.5 according to the moral constructs that I'm proposing in this book—vigilance, mindfulness, compliance, and humility:

Vigilance: Assume that vigilance refers to cognitive acts or behaviors that continuously monitor the external physical environment for hazard opportunities. As such, the startling aspect of Case 1.5 is the staff's failure to notice that the ventilator wasn't engaged for a significant period during the operation. Yet, the literature on medical error is replete with instances wherein personnel are inattentive to where danger or error opportunities lurk—not because they are careless or stupid, but because they are not practiced or sensitive in gauging or anticipating the level of threat.[34(pp26-63)] A central component of professionals' vigilant orientation is exercising their "foreseeability," whereby they are keenly aware of the likely consequences of the unique operator-to-environment interface.[24] But the human nervous system does not allow us to be sharply attentive and vigilant every second of our waking hours, so complex systems such as those in healthcare are often supplemented with safety devices or technologies that compensate for the imperfections of human performance. In hindsight, then, disabling the monitoring and alarm system in the operating room seems an extraordinarily incautious decision and a moral lapse.

Mindfulness: If vigilance connotes a monitoring of the external environment for threats, then mindfulness connotes monitoring one's internal or psychological environment for cognitive lapses that can imperil patient safety. Distractions are extremely common in error commission, and we see them in this case.[35] Were it not for the equipment failures of the operating room table and the x-ray machine, the anesthesiologist's mindful attentiveness might not have been disrupted. Over the years of discussing this case, anesthesiologists have told me that when they turn off a ventilator, one technique they use to remind themselves to turn it back on is to keep a finger on the toggle switch or to take a deep breath and hold it until they turn the ventilator back on. Failing to do these things while the operating room's alarms were disengaged put the anesthesiologist at the mercy of his imperfect sensory and attentional equipment, which failed to register the harm that was developing just a few feet away.

Noncompliance: Health professionals are expected to comply with rules, regulations, and standards. While I never learned this with certainty, it would not have been unusual if the mechanical problems with the operating room table and the x-ray machine had previously occurred. A recurring theme in patient safety is how often staff members are aware of workflow and environmental problems and noncompliance but call no attention to them. Usually, personnel are able to work around or compensate for such problems, which many prefer to do as they fear retaliation for pointing out an operational (or operator) problem. Of course, had the anesthesiologist simply remembered to turn the ventilator back on, the anoxic disaster would likely not have occurred despite malfunctioning technology. But how would patient safety leadership receive the idea of disabling the alarms in the operating room? Notice how multiple factors, like a lack of vigilance, poor compliance, and attentional disruptions can mix and result in disaster. Another sad fact, however, is that such "resident pathogens," as one scholar called them, are always present in any complex system.[1(p197)] They cannot be entirely removed; hence, because no environment is perfectly safe, whatever one can reasonably do to maintain vigilance, mindfulness, and compliance will enhance patient safety.

Humility: None of the personnel taking care of Mrs. Smith ever told her family about the ventilator error. At the anesthesiologist's deposition, he explained that he couldn't be "one hundred percent certain" that the anoxic event caused the patient's chronic unconsciousness, so he felt that the causational component of Mrs. Smith's anoxia could not justly be characterized as negligence on his part. The surgeon responded that he felt horrible about what happened, but that this was the anesthesiologist's error, not his, so it was up to the anesthesiologist to confess what happened. The hospital, in turn, had no policy for disclosing an error when the attending physicians refused to. At this point, the case recalls some traditional bioethical maxims on accommodating a family's right to information (which was ignored by the error concealment), as well as highlighting how error concealment caused additional suffering to the family by dismissing their questions about what caused their mother's demise. By way of "explanation," the surgeon told the family that their mother must have had an intra- or a postoperative stroke, which the surgeon rationalized as "truthful" since strokes include anoxic events. Under the circumstances, many persons would likely consider that a frank dissimulation, and the family members related in their depositions that they had suspected early on that critical information was being withheld. It seems fair to say that the healthcare team could not find the requisite humility along with the moral courage to disclose the ventilator error, such that when the family did find out, they felt betrayed and proceeded to sue. One might also argue that disabling the alarm system in the operating room was a foolhardy act of overconfidence given any operating room staff's limited attentional capacity.

Comparing the Cases

Traditional ethical thinking and analysis is typically concerned with articulating the most compelling and persuasive strategy or resolution for a case like 1.4. These situations sometimes bewilder us because they can occur without precedent, so we feel we are without a moral compass to guide us to a resolution. That absence of precedents often derives from a case being complicated by its biotechnology, such as the complexity of modern operating rooms equipped with machines that can assume the patient's vital organ functioning even when he or she is declared "dead."

While Case 1.4 is analytically complex because of numerous principle-based considerations at hand, Case 1.5 is frankly horrifying, owing to the multiple imperfections in the human-to-environment encounter. Whether to engage a ventilator that has been left off for an inordinate amount of time is not a recondite decision. Failure to do so is an inarguable performance error resulting from the imperfections of human cognition and its performance environment. Thus, whereas the typical bioethics case is one that seeks a principled or theoretically based resolution informed by a group's understanding of rightness and goodness, the patient safety case of 1.5 is much more performatively oriented and looks to the practice policies, requirements, and obligations that all professionals should exercise in providing patients with reasonably safe environments. Put otherwise, the typical bioethics dilemma might involve various principles or constructs bearing on individual rights, harms, benefits, and fairness to solve puzzles over a moral agent's rights or obligations. Patient safety ethics, however, targets only one moral objective: to mitigate as much as possible performance-based and environmental factors that threaten patient safety.

This is not to say that patient safety ethics examines only the perceptual, cognitive, or attitudinal missteps of health professionals or the error traps of their environments. Fundamental philosophical concepts like acceptable risk, standard of care, the nature of error, and many more that I discuss in this book require the analytical tools of traditional bioethical thinking and analysis. Nevertheless, patient safety ethics diverges from the clinical bioethics tradition in the more rule-driven, attentively oriented, risk-conscious, and self-monitoring demands of delivering healthcare, rather than the more contemplative, value-driven, and dilemmatic nature of bioethical challenges that require a thoughtful and sensitive resolution.

Conclusion

This first chapter discusses certain foundational ethical constructs that inform and shape patient safety. At the heart of these discussions lies the question of the nature and extent of a professional's obligation in matters of patient safety. No environment is perfectly safe, and all human beings are fallible. Complex systems never run perfectly and will frequently pose unanticipated or unprecedented navigational challenges to system operators. The care process can be enormously complex such that a modest error or mistake can occur at any step and cause disaster down the road. The challenge this presents requires developing an attitudinal and performative skill set that, at its core, involves safety wisdom being attained and exercised among all health professionals. Acquiring this knowledge and skill set is not easy, especially as it invites the challenge, discussed in the next chapter, of cultivating and sharpening the first of four dimensions of error wisdom: vigilance.

2 Vigilance

Safety management must also be proactive, so that interventions are made before something happens and can affect how it will happen or even prevent something from happening.

Erik Hollnagel, Robert L. Wears, and Jeffrey Braithwaite[1(p21)]

Chapter Overview: This chapter is divided into two parts. Part I offers a conceptual overview of vigilance, foreseeability, and their roles in developing the skill set of a reasonably cautious person. The work of Danish errorologist Erik Hollnagel is featured, as Hollnagel encourages patient safety expertise to be directed away from a singular focus on errors and toward appreciating the improvisatory powers of skillful health professionals who maintain patient safety despite the ubiquity of hazard pitfalls and error threats. I largely argue that the skill set Hollnagel applauds is a critical component of vigilance. Part II of the chapter focuses on the nature of harm: How harm might be understood from within an ethical framework; how harming someone can differ from wronging the person; and how to determine ethically "acceptable" risks of harm in a particular context, considering that risk will always exist in every environment to some degree. The chapter concludes with some practical manifestations of vigilance that token the reasonably cautious person, followed by an interview of Richard Cook, who supports Hollnagel's position and offers additional and somewhat iconoclastic insights.

PART I: VIGILANCE, FORESEEABILITY, AND THE REASONABLY CAUTIOUS PERSON

Characterizing Vigilance

Psychiatrist Glen Gabbard has opined, "There is no doubt that compulsiveness is the hallmark of the physician's personality," adding that "compulsive traits are present in the majority of those individuals who seek out medicine as a career."[2(p2926)] I am unaware of any empirical data to back up Gabbard's claims, but patients obviously want their physicians to leave no reasonable diagnostic or treatment-related stones unturned. If health professionals are to refrain from committing harm from error, they must be attentive to and perhaps at least somewhat "compulsive" about recognizing the harm opportunities that threaten patients, and then be persistent in eliminating or defusing these threats.

Given the pathological connotations of "compulsive," though, perhaps a better word is "vigilant"—which the *Oxford Living Dictionaries* defines as "the action or state of keeping careful watch for possible danger or difficulties."[3] Clearly, vigilance is critical to patient safety as its absence is so often implicated in catastrophes and headline-grabbing medical malpractice cases. In one such case in 2003, 13-year-old Jesica Santillan received a heart-lung transplant from a donor whose organ blood type (A) didn't match hers (O+), a fact that multiple health professionals missed.[4] An earlier case, in 1995, involved a prize-winning *Boston Globe* columnist, Betsy Lehman, who was to receive 1,630 mg of a potent chemotherapeutic drug (cyclophosphamide) daily for four days. Instead, she received the four-day total, 6,520 mg, *per day*, causing her death. Lois Ayash, the leader of Lehman's care team, told the *New York Times*, "It was a blunder compounded or overlooked by at least a dozen physicians, nurses and pharmacists, including some of the institution's senior staff."[5]

Similarly, I was involved in the situation briefly described as Case 1.2 in the previous chapter, in which too many clinicians failed to notice that their patient had been receiving a 16-fold overdose, for two days, of a drug called acetylcysteine, which is used to protect the liver from acetaminophen overdoses. Here's a more detailed account of what happened to this patient, whom I'll call Lily, and the aftermath:

Case 2.1. Lily mistakenly and unintentionally ingested too much Tylenol and became ill. On arriving at a local hospital's emergency room, her ER physician elected to treat the overdose with a drug called acetylcysteine (Acetadote). The medicine is delivered intravenously over a 21-hour period, and Lily should have received a total of about 480 mL of the medicine (or about half of a one-liter bag). The ER physician had never ordered acetylcysteine before, however, and the original order sent to the pharmacy was incomplete and incorrect. The pharmacist who filled the order had never dispensed acetylcysteine either, but he spotted the physician's erroneous order and rewrote it. His revision contained the 16-fold dosing error. The pharmacist physically took his rewritten order to the ER physician, who signed it without checking its accuracy. The physician would later assert that because pharmacists are the experts, she felt it unnecessary to check their work. The infusion nurse who would calibrate the infusion pump had never infused acetylcysteine before. She looked up information about the drug in a formulary and printed a copy of the dosing instructions, which she placed in Lily's chart, but the nurse failed to study the instructions that she had looked up or to compare them to the written order. Instead, she set the flow pump exactly as the order dictated and later claimed at her deposition that this was all the nursing standard of care required her to do.

The hospitalist physician who later admitted Lily was also unfamiliar with acetylcysteine, but hospital protocol stipulated that on transfer, all drugs be discontinued and new medication orders written. The hospitalist, who later said that she had been unaware of this rule, ordered that the acetylcysteine be continued at the original, mistaken dosage.

Lily received the 16-fold overdose of acetylcysteine for about 35 of the approximately 55 hours she spent in the hospital. (There were many delays in replacing the bags each time one emptied, which happened rapidly at the inflated infusion rate.) So instead of the half bag Lily would have gone through in total at the correct dosage, her healthcare team ended up ordering six bags from the pharmacy over the next two days, which caused the pharmacy, in turn, to order 14 boxes of acetylcysteine from a supplier. Although such high use of the drug was extremely unusual, no one called attention to it. And even though pharmacy policy stated that at the end of a medication regimen, new orders for a drug needed to be written, Lily's physicians—with one exception—continued the original, erroneous order. Strangely, by the end of the first 21-hour administration, Lily's acetaminophen level was 10 mcg/ml, which no longer required acetylcysteine. Approximately 90 minutes later, however, another physician ordered that the latter drug be continued for another 18 hours.

Approximately 20 hours into her hospital stay, Lily was noted to be "sluggish." A few hours later, she became agitated, arguably demonstrating an altered mental state. Despite hospital policy, Lily's nurse did not contact a physician. About 12 hours later, and as her mental status continued to deteriorate, Lily pulled out her IV—an ironic moment—and the nurse called the physician. Contrary to protocol, the physician did not evaluate Lily's altered mental status but ordered a "straight push" of 5 mg of Haldol, which lowers seizure threshold. Within 5 minutes, Lily began having seizures, which would continue uncontrolled for the next 4 hours. The nurse on duty called Lily's physician and later claimed to have called a rapid response team that she said appeared, but no documentation attests to the team's appearance, and no member of the rapid response team self-identified as having treated Lily. In fact, there were no nurse's notes during this 4-hour period, so it remained unknown what kind of treatment Lily actually received, if any. Lily's (night/early morning) physician never saw her during the 4-hour uncontrolled seizure period but instead managed her care over the phone. Even though this physician had responsibility for Lily over her 12-hour shift, during which time the seizures began, and then the following evening for about 6 hours, she never saw or examined her patient during the entirety of Lily's hospitalization.

Lily was seen and examined by a daytime staff physician, but he was also unfamiliar with acetylcysteine and gave a telephonic order for its 18-hour administration, which a nurse retrieving the call recorded at the 16-fold overdose rate. Lily began receiving this second round of medicine around 10 am. This would essentially be a *new* order and subject to review and check by the pharmacy—but that apparently did not occur. Pharmacy staff would later contend that it was a "continuation" of the previous order. At 7 pm that (second) night—and 9 hours into the 18-hour/16-fold overdose order—the medicine had run out and a fresh bag needed to be hung. Two hours elapsed before this happened, but when the bag was hung around 9 pm, the nurse reset the flow rate from the 16-fold overdose rate to an acceptable one. Amazingly, she made this change without a physician's order. A nurse ordinarily cannot unilaterally change the medication or its dose. But she did. At deposition, the nurse claimed she had no memory of how this happened, so the dosing change went unexplained.

Lily was discharged to another hospital about 6 hours later. Soon after her admission, her brain herniated, leaving her in a vegetative state from which she has never recovered. The hospital that overdosed Lily charged her family more than $15,000 for the acetylcysteine that was used during the course of her care. Part of the high charge was the cost of the emergency reorders the pharmacy had to do. Although the pharmacy department apparently received reports calling attention to the elevated usage, no policy or procedure was in place to check on or monitor such unusual occurrences. The case settled out of court for $15.5 million.

James Reason believes that "omissions are likely to be the single most frequent error type,"[6(p32)] an observation that speaks directly to the challenge of maintaining vigilance. Case 2.1 is a tragic example. The fundamental problem that permeates this case seemed to be the staff's unfamiliarity with administering acetylcysteine according to the 21-hour protocol. Absent that knowledge, it was virtually impossible for them to know *what to be vigilant about.* Obviously, any of them would instantly question an order for a patient to be given 100 mg of oxycodone or 100 units of insulin. But no one seemed familiar with a safe dose of acetylcysteine, which was then followed by subsequent vigilance failures: Everyone assumed the ER physician's order (as rewritten by the pharmacist) was correct. The ER physician didn't check the pharmacist's order; the infusion nurse likewise trusted the order, as did the hospitalist who admitted Lily to the floor. Furthermore, multiple pharmacists refilled the overdose order, amounting to several bags of medicine, but never checked the order's accuracy. Notice that even if rules, regulations, standards, and policies are in place to vigilantly maintain patient safety, failing to comply with them will inject excessive laxity into the system, which jeopardizes safety.

The hospitalist's failure to visit and evaluate Lily, much less attend to her progressively deteriorating condition, may arguably amount to malpractice, but the change in dosage to an acceptable amount by the nurse absent a physician's order seems perfectly bizarre. When I chatted with some nurse friends about this, they hypothesized that the nurse might have contacted the attending physician, who could have told her to adjust the flow rate properly, but if so, the nurse then neglected to document the conversation as a verbal order. A more chilling hypothesis is that the nurse may have been explicitly told not to document the order as a new one. Still another possibility is that the nurse just took it on herself to change the flow rate without telling the attending physician, which would have been a gross violation of the nursing standard of care. I do know, however, that the plaintiffs in this case had experts prepared to testify that someone at the hospital had figured out that Lily was being overdosed and had then tried to prevent the overdose from being discovered.

This case stands as a remarkable example of how, beginning with a lack of familiarity with a care intervention involving an intravenous drug, the operational defenses of an otherwise modern and technologically sophisticated hospital can fail and end in tragedy. Multiple staff members frankly didn't know where risks and harms resided—among themselves, within their work environment, or in the intervention requirements—so they couldn't orient their vigilance accurately. How, then, might patient safety efforts better teach and internalize an attitude and practice of vigilance?

Vigilance, Foreseeability, and the Reasonably Cautious Person

Assuming the truth of Gabbard's remark that compulsiveness is a hallmark of the physician's personality—which, he recently informed me, he continues to staunchly believe—the question arises whether vigilant individuals are born that way or develop compulsiveness in their training. Because medical students are typically academic superstars, I suspect that many are compulsive learners. They know how to study; they appreciate what's important to know; they're good at seeing conceptual connections and relationships as well as their underlying logic; they are willing to put in long hours studying and learning; and they have fabulous memories. These traits serve them well when they meet up with the rigors of medical training, which has been wryly described as "learning to drink water from a fire hose."[7] Importantly, though, the bare thought of seriously harming a patient by error must be acutely anxiety provoking to these intelligent and well-intentioned learners (and to veteran clinicians as well), such that it is easy to see how Gabbard's thesis on compulsiveness—understood as a defense mechanism against the possibility of error commission—is highly plausible.

Still, such compulsiveness must be shaped and directed by the right kind of knowledge; a physician might be compulsive about scheduling patients for yearly physicals but poor at performing them, for example, or compulsive about having the latest technology but careless in learning how to use it properly. Alternatively, physicians exquisitely compulsive about their performance could be uncaring or indifferent toward the competence of their colleagues.

In the penultimate chapter of Reason's *The Human Contribution*, he describes vigilant, error-sharpened individuals in terms of their (1) comprehensive understanding of how the system works, especially in knowing where to look, what to expect, and what action plans to launch when things malfunction; (2) acceptance of the fact that errors can and will occur; (3) knowledge of where particular pitfalls lie *before beginning a task*; (4) contingency plans to deal with anticipated problems; (5) readiness to seek help (along with a keen appreciation of when they are over their head); (6) careful evaluation and wariness of colleagues' knowledge and experience, "especially when they are strangers"; and (7) skepticism toward assumptions, which can lead to disaster by persuading health professionals that they need not check and recheck.[6] Reason's heroes are personnel who experience "a chronic unease, or the continual expectation that things can and will go wrong," and who foster

> a reporting culture by commending, even rewarding, people for reporting their errors and close calls. They work on the assumption that what seems to be an isolated failure is likely to come from the confluence of many upstream contributing factors. Instead of localizing failures, they generalize them. Instead of applying local repairs, they strive for system reforms. They do not take the past as an infallible guide to the future. Aware that system failures can take a variety of yet-to-be-encountered forms, they are continually on the lookout for "sneak paths" or novel ways in which active failures and latent conditions can combine to defeat or by-pass the defences, barriers and safeguards. In short, collectively mindful organisations are preoccupied with the possibility of failure . . . [T]hey appear to maintain high levels of chronic unease and a twitchy vigilance.[6(p259)]

This is a marvelous characterization of vigilance and, by extension, the reasonably cautious health professional. The ethical aspects of patient safety are decidedly performative, epistemic, and attitudinal. Vigilance, experience, and hazard awareness help professionals recognize and halt harm opportunities that lurk in their midst. If the hero of classical bioethics is the brilliant analyst who can dissect a complex moral situation into its abstract parts and resolve their tensions with a principled based set of suggestions, then the patient safety hero is the reasonably cautious person—Reason's agent of "twitchy vigilance"—who maintains a keen risk evaluation of the work environment and is ready to snuff out error opportunities and hazard pitfalls.

Foreseeability

Part of vigilant practice is exercising foresight, or foreseeability, which Reason describes as "the ability to identify, respond to, and recover from the initial indications that a patient safety incident could take place."[6(p250)] Throughout this book, vigilance connotes monitoring the *external* practice environment (in contrast to mindfulness, which refers to monitoring one's *internal* cognitive and emotional environment). Tort law, which takes seriously the concept of foreseeability, has defined it to include "risks that an actor may not know but reasonably should, commonly explained in constructive knowledge terms as risks the actor 'should have known,' meaning that prudence sometimes requires actors to investigate and evaluate possibilities of hidden or inchoate risk."[8(p1292)]

Vigilance, foreseeability, and the reasonably cautious person are overlapping and self-reinforcing notions that help determine an individual's responsibility for a harm occurrence. If the harm a patient experienced was reasonably preventable, then we would indict that person's care providers for their lack of vigilance or caution. But if the harmful event was unpredictable, perhaps the result of an unusually complex or eccentric chain of causation that no reasonable health professional could have anticipated and managed, then we can hardly criticize the healthcare provider for lacking foreseeability. Again, the reasonably cautious person will, among other things, persistently direct a critical look at his or her performance environment's imperfections and their potential for harm. Consider this example:

Case 2.2. A heavily sedated female patient was placed in a holding room in the psychiatric unit of a hospital to await the availability of a bed. Two male psychiatric patients were also in the holding unit. The video monitor in that room clearly showed one of the men sexually molesting the woman multiple times, although he would first glance out the window of the room to the nurses' station to make sure that no staff would likely enter while he committed the rapes. Each attack lasted less than a minute. When the woman reported the attacks, and the video feed provided proof of them, the holding room was remodeled, presumably to allow greater visual access and protection of patients. The case settled out of court.

After disasters like this occur, how they could and should have been prevented becomes painfully obvious to staff. But while the harm opportunity was present, no one took the initiative, or exercised foreseeability, to enact measures that would have prevented the injurious event, suggesting a lack of foreseeability that can be damning in medical malpractice cases.

I recently consulted on three rape cases in psychiatric hospitals where some or all of the following variables causally contributed to the plaintiffs' allegations:

- Male and female patients were allowed to commingle in their care environments.
- The nurses' station had poor visualization, or "blind spots," to certain areas of the unit.

- Video monitoring was either nonexistent or was used only for forensic, after-the-fact investigations; it was not used to prevent or mitigate the threat of sexual attacks.
- If video monitoring was present on the unit, staff members were unsure whether they were supposed to be monitoring the video feed in real time; alternatively, they confessed to not having a policy that would clarify the unit's video-monitoring practices.
- Certain safety policies—such as one facility's mandate that doors to patients' rooms remain open—were not enforced.
- The customary 15-minute staff check on psychiatric patients was infrequently performed and, in any case, proved insufficient to deter the would-be rapist.[9]

In the immediate aftermath of these attacks, certain involved staff members were as stunned as they were saddened. They expressed astonishment that such a thing could happen on their units and, in two of the cases, argued that they had done nothing wrong despite compelling evidence of the rapes. These defendants seemed to suffer from impoverished imaginations that prevented their appreciating the risks to which their patients were exposed. Yet, we must grant the possibility that in some instances, staff members do exercise reasonable caution and foreseeability, yet an adverse event happens anyway. In those situations, we cannot ascribe negligence to them because they acted sensibly and maintained environments that were "reasonably" safe. Even so, the hindsight bias is so powerful that when a sexual attack occurs, courts are likely to hold treating professionals to a high level of accountability and foreseeability.

Vigilance: On Things Usually Going Right

My interview with Richard Cook at the end of this chapter offers an interesting and important perspective on how vigilance might be understood in a somewhat nontraditional way. In the interview, Cook approvingly mentions the work of Erik Hollnagel, who, along with Robert Wears and Jeffrey Braithwaite, published a paper, *From Safety-I to Safety-II: A White Paper*, that offers an overview of the kind of safety considerations and understandings that Cook encourages.[1] The important point is that things usually go right because health professionals know how to accommodate their behaviors to a constantly changing and oftentimes chaotic work environment, which would be impossible if the staff didn't practice vigilance.

Hollnagel believes that our traditional approach to patient safety, perhaps best represented by the root cause analyses with which hospital risk managers are so familiar, needs to be complemented (although not replaced) by another approach. The traditional view, which Hollnagel terms "Safety-I," understands safety as "the prevention of errors and adverse effects to patients associated with health care."[1(p6)] In this account, preventable adverse events are largely explained by cause and effect relations, and they are decomposable; that is, they can be isolated or partitioned off from the normal event flow and studied as atomistic-like happenings or photograph-like snapshots. Safety-I analyses proceed by detecting the malfunctions that cause safety lapses so that we can fix them. A system that works well is one that functions as the system architects imagined it would. A system that works poorly is one that witnesses accidents owing to malfunctions or abnormalities, often resulting from noncompliance with regulations or standards. Safety-I systems are therefore understood bimodally; that is, they either function correctly or not, with adversities representing a proxy for safety: the smaller the number of preventable adverse events, the safer the system. Safety, then, is defined in Safety-I by the prevalence of its opposite: harm. Vigilance doesn't much enter Hollnagel's Safety-I characterization as its role is largely subsumed by rule or standard-of-care adherence.

In contrast to this traditional view of safety, Hollnagel and his colleagues propose another model, which Richard Cook endorses in our interview. This view, termed "Safety-II," understands work environments as inherently dynamic, unstable, intractable, unpredictable, too fluid to be decomposable, and replete with system operators constantly making tweaks and adjustments that, more often than not, enable their performance goals to be accomplished. Whereas Safety-I emphasizes safety from the perspective of mistakes and errors, Safety-II emphasizes safety as learning from all the things *that are going right*. Safety-II is immensely impressed when "doctors, nurses and allied health staff perform safely because they are able to adjust their work so that it matches the conditions."[1(p17)] The reason for such work adjustments is that health professionals have little choice: their task environments are often frantic, chaotic, unpredictable, frenzied, and fraught with high emotions that can upset objective reasoning. Still, most of the time things go swimmingly, which is what impresses Hollnagel and his colleagues: Why, in the midst of remarkable flux and unpredictability, do system operators witness so few disasters? What do they do that seems so abundantly right? Under this view, then, what is the content of their "vigilance"?

Vigilance in Safety-II

I find Hollnagel's emphasis on things going right and the necessity of practice variation to enable safety as requiring a *deeper kind* of vigilance than that of the Safety-I system operator. The latter, I believe, takes a rather static perspective on safety and understands it as threatened when standard operating procedures are violated or when recognized hazard pitfalls are allowed to persist or go unquestioned in the performance environment. Hollnagel would certainly concur that such behavior imperils safety, but his Safety-II platform implicates a notion of vigilance more characteristic of a veteran professional—perhaps of the type Reason described—whose ability to safely "go with the flow" reveals a deep hazard awareness because the practice environment is susceptible to change at a moment's notice. Likely, then, this individual will want to ensure that hazard pitfalls are eliminated as much as possible *to begin with* so that they do not invite unnecessary risk at a later point when the unexpected occurs. Thus, it seems inevitable that this person would utilize some Safety-I methods.

Still, and as much as I admire Hollnagel's account and believe it resonates nicely with the representation of vigilance on offer here, I want to take issue with some of his insights, especially that situations evade decomposability and that errors as causes are often hard to detect and can arouse bitter disagreement. Consider this "medical misadventure":

Case 2.3. The patient was admitted to the hospital for a laparoscopically assisted vaginal hysterectomy. Because she'd already had multiple abdominal surgeries, a laparoscopic approach might not have been the best clinical decision, but the matter is debatable and is certainly subject to hindsight bias. After a few hours in surgery, the gynecological surgeon decided he could not complete the procedure laparoscopically, so he converted to a laparotomy, that is, an open procedure, and was able to successfully remove the patient's uterus.

Because the procedure changed from a closed to an open surgery, representing what the hospital calls an "emergent circumstance," an intraoperative x-ray was required, at least to ensure that no foreign bodies were retained. At that point, the circulating nurse had charted the sponge count as being 10 of 10 and informed the surgeon. Nevertheless, a radio-opaque laparotomy pad was left in the patient's lower right quadrant.

The hospital's policies and procedures require that the intraoperative x-ray be sent to a radiologist, who reads and reports his or her findings directly back to the surgical suite. The x-ray was taken and sent; however, the scan was erroneously marked REGULAR rather than URGENT, and therefore by the time it was read, the surgeon had begun another procedure. Furthermore, the radiologist misidentified the lap pad as a drain. The surgeon claimed in his deposition that if the scan had been processed earlier, he would have likely remembered that there was no drain in place, and presumably he would have re-entered the patient's abdomen and searched for a retained object.

The hospital's policies and procedures clearly state that a patient is not to be removed from the surgical suite until the radiologist has spoken *directly* with the circulating nurse or the surgeon by phone. Although the testimony is conflicting, the surgeon may have never received the radiologist's report. The physician did testify, however, that while he was dictating his surgical notes in the adjoining room and waiting for the radiologic report, he had looked up to see the circulating nurse removing the patient and giving him a thumbs up. He had taken that to mean that the patient was cleared, that is, that the radiologic report had come back and indicated nothing unusual. The circulating nurse asserted in her testimony that the surgeon had become impatient waiting to hear from radiology and had simply instructed the staff to take the patient to recovery.

The patient was discharged home with the retained laparotomy pad. Also, at some point during her surgery, her bowel had been damaged such that when she returned to the hospital three days after discharge, she had a temperature of 103.6 degrees Fahrenheit, a pulse between 122 and 137, an elevated white blood cell count, and complaints of terrible abdominal pain, vaginal bleeding, and anorexia. Although the surgeon ordered a CT scan of her abdomen, a series of delays followed, ultimately postponing the scan until the next morning. Plaintiff's counsel was ready to produce experts who would testify that these delays were marked by a failure to appreciate how ill the patient was, poor or nonexistent hand-off communications among the nurses, and, at least according to one expert witness, an absence of proper advocacy for the patient. The following morning, the patient went into cardiac arrest and was anoxic or hypoxic for about 14 minutes. When the surgical team opened her abdomen, they observed about 2,500 ml of fecal matter, which had seeped in from the laceration to her sigmoid colon. The patient expired 3 weeks later.

Although Hollnagel argues against the "decomposability" of error events, it seems perfectly acceptable to isolate moments of error in this case, especially the mislabeled scan (REGULAR rather than URGENT), the omitted communication between the radiologist and the surgeon, and the decision to transport the patient to recovery before receiving the scan results. Hospital risk management would surely want to investigate each of these lapses and implement system changes, perhaps reminiscent of a Safety-I approach, intended to prevent recurrence of similar mistakes. Yet, these errors amounted to far more than "performance variation." All errors—if we understand them as deviations from the standard of care—are variations, but in situations like this one, where the outcome is catastrophic, error as "variation" seems to ignore the gravity of the patient's condition, the harm she experienced, and what standard-of-care judgment might encourage. A case like this one demonstrates that paying attention to what goes right will not be helpful when multiple events concatenate and result in disaster. Of course, the performance adjustments that Hollnagel discussed are indeed worth examining in the majority of instances when things go well, and they are no doubt integral to an attitude of vigilance. But these adjustments seem entirely out of place when errors due to vigilance lapses contaminate those performance variations and doom the outcome. Furthermore, to comprehend "going well" with an interpretive eye to "going poorly" seems only logical. Neither term appears to have meaningful content without an appreciation of the other.

Nevertheless, this case illustrates several points on which Hollnagel, Cook, and I entirely concur, such as how performance pressures alter customary safety practices in favor of "efficiency." Clearly, production quotas were weighing heavily on the judgment of both the physician and the circulating nurse, and neither had any reason to believe that the surgery had gone poorly when the patient was removed to the recovery room. As Cook points out in his interview, production pressures militate against vigilance, since the latter sometimes requires an extended and concentrated block of time, which production pressures might discourage.

Consider Hollnagel's belief that Safety-I and Safety-II "represent two complementary views of safety rather than two incompatible or conflicting approaches,"[1(p26)] and that "the way ahead lies not in a replacement of Safety-I by Safety-II, but rather in a combination of the two ways of thinking."[1(p30)] An emphasis on things going wrong is decidedly different from Hollnagel's, but perhaps both approaches ultimately and simultaneously alight on what he stresses as "an overall comprehensive view of work . . .

[which involves] [b]eing sensitive to what happens, to the ways in which it can succeed as well as the ways in which it can fail."[1(p29)] This is vigilance in a nutshell. Part II of this chapter presents some strategies for realizing that comprehensive view of work.

PART II: VIGILANCE, HARM, AND RISK

In intrinsically hazardous systems, operators are expected to encounter and appreciate hazards in ways that lead to overall performance that is desirable. Improved safety depends on providing operators with calibrated views of the hazards. It also depends on providing calibration about how their actions move system performance towards or away from the edge of the [hazard] envelope.

Richard Cook[10(p4)]

The Threat of Harm in Healthcare Environments

Health professionals know that they are obligated by ethical codes as well as by accreditation standards not only to refrain from causing harm but to provide patients with reasonably safe environments, that is, environments where the risk of harm is "acceptable." Obviously, translating patient safety into the language of harm seems eminently reasonable, because if no harms could ever occur to patients, *there would be nothing patients needed to be protected from and nothing health professionals would need to be vigilant about.* Safety therefore implies enjoying some acceptable but relative (rather than absolute) degree of protection from a harm occurrence.[1] Importantly, then, safety can be thought of as an emergent property resulting from health professionals doing things correctly, which, as I'm arguing in this book, occurs from practicing vigilance, mindfulness, compliance, and humility.

Harm avoidance is hard wired into our neural circuitry. Neuroevolution has equipped our brains with plenty of resources to attend to and to avoid harm, such as attention-focusing programs like feelings and emotions that rivet attention on potential dangers, memory capabilities that enable us to recall dangerous or menacing experiences, and a remarkable readiness to activate defensive or protective (motor- and neuroendocrine-based) behavioral responses, like RUN AWAY!, when confronted with apparent menace or peril.[11]

But these are all examples of avoiding harm to oneself, not refraining from harming others. A common worry in patient safety, as illustrated in Case 2.1, is how ordinarily well-meaning, competent health professionals are sometimes oblivious to the threats, hazards, and risks that not only lurk in their work environments, but that they themselves enable. Their sensitivity to the possibility of harm seems blunted by numerous factors, such as production pressures, which encourage risk taking; a lack of knowledge about harm possibilities, which contributes to carelessness; and elements of the work atmosphere, especially the physical environment and its associated technologies, that compound the potential hazards in their surroundings.[12] Herbert Simon dubbed this tripartite matrix of limitations—compromised cognition, knowledge, and environment—"bounded rationality," a construct that permeates the narratives of this book.[13]

Not only would patient safety ethics be nonexistent without harm probabilities and materialization, but bioethics and ethical theory would be lost without harms. Perhaps there would continue to be a need for ethical theories on improving the quality of the human experience or human happiness, but even these interests seem motivated by the threat of harm, the potential for a suboptimal quality of life, or simply the menacing possibility of undesirable happenings. What is unassailable, however, is that the significance of theoretical and practical concern over the nature and risk of harm materialization is a mainstay in patient safety and medical ethics.[14(p154)]

Patient safety and the need for vigilance are conditioned by the inevitability, familiarity, unpredictability, and undesirability of harm. Depending on how we define harm—especially if we adopt Joel Feinberg's famous characterization of it as a "setback of interest"—patients are harmed not only by suffering from uncomfortable programs of care, but by having to take time off from work, spend money to drive to a clinic or hospital, find a parking place, and wait an uncomfortably long time to see a health professional.[15] Yet, most healthcare providers would not assume any responsibility for these latter kinds of "harms," which are caused by factors beyond their control. The harms that should concern health professionals are the *reasonably preventable* ones within their sphere of control and responsibility, that is, the ones that any reasonable health professional would take steps to avert or fend off.[16] Indeed, a clinician's failure to take measures to protect patients from a reasonably preventable harm that then materialized would count as not just harming patients but *wronging* them.[17] In other words, healthcare consumers have a right to receive care that accords with the professional standard and that is delivered safely. When that right is disappointed, as in most of the cases described in this book, the patient has been wronged.

A Troubling Variable: The Cost of Risk Reduction

A disturbing fact of life is that the level of safety we enjoy is often a function of what we can economically afford. The economics of risk—which is a cost estimate of harm relative to its probability and magnitude compared to the relative costs required to reduce its likelihood—permeates our existence, from the foods we eat, the cars we drive, and the jobs we work to the homes and neighborhoods we reside in, the entertainment we enjoy, and the company we keep.[6(pp230-37)] In healthcare, the correlation between higher risk of harm and less ability to pay is well documented according to measures like increased infant mortality, longer waits to be seen in clinics and hospitals, insurance coverage exclusions, shorter hospital stays, poorer overall health, and heightened risk of death.[18]

The question that now confronts us is the degree of risk patients might be subjected to, especially if different patients might be exposed to disparate levels of safety. Although access to healthcare may well be a function of economic factors, *all* patients in a given clinic or hospital should enjoy the same level of safety. But this doesn't always happen, as illustrated in the next case:

Case 2.4. In the late 1970s and early '80s, a respected academic eye center allegedly scheduled eye surgeries based on patients' financial means, with wellheeled, well-insured patients invariably receiving appointments early in the day, followed by those with less and less coverage and ability to pay as the day progressed. By day's end, patients without insurance were having their surgeries. This was claimed to be standard policy, which, if true, meant that the poor were more likely to be operated on by possibly fatigued surgeons and therefore bore a heightened risk of injury. Toward the end of one particular day in surgery, a patient with poor reimbursement had an operation on the wrong eye. Admission of the error was initially withheld.[19]

Many persons would denounce this scheduling practice as discriminatory. If patient-centered care is a fundamental ethical construct in contemporary medicine, then the practice described above seems an affront to human dignity by systematically exposing a particular group of persons to an elevated degree of risk. Yet, one can imagine economists of the Hayek-Friedman camp not having a problem with this arrangement at all. Although poorer patients' risk exposure in this example would incontestably be elevated in comparison to well-insured, financially secure patients, some ideologues (especially those who espouse a marketplace platform for understanding justice and the distribution of social goods) might argue that for poorer patients, receiving a valuable service, namely, the restoration of their vision, without charge is an acceptable trade-off. Although that risk was never disclosed to these less well-off patients, as ethics would demand it be, many might conceivably accept the risk in return for free eye surgery.

Of course, a clinician cannot waive his or her legal liability, as in "I'll operate on you for free, Mr. Jones, if you promise not to sue me if anything goes wrong." Everyone has a right to safe care regardless of means, so any patients in Case 2.4 who were harmed by an exhausted physician's negligence would have the right to recover damages, which is what happened. The more trenchant problem is that risks fluctuate from patient to patient and hospital to hospital for all sorts of reasons, such as the patient's ability to pay; the staff's level of training; the hospital's economic resources, whereby it can purchase the latest technologies and attract and retain highly skilled and well-motivated personnel; the administration's insistence on efficiency (which can compromise safety); and the fact that some hospitals cater to a wealthier and healthier population, who can maintain their health better and access good healthcare faster than their less well-off counterparts.[20] Consequently, agreeing on an ethically acceptable level of risk turns out to be challenging because it is beset by certain system variables that affect risk variation and fluctuation. If vigilance is an ethically significant construct in patient safety ethics, then risk or hazard awareness must be objectively discernible and manageable; otherwise vigilance will have no meaningful content or direction.

Criteria of Risk Acceptability

Determining which risks in life are acceptable and which ones not rests on deciding what criteria or principles will inform those determinations. In chapter 6, I argue, and supplement with a case example, that (1) the continuum of risk probability and severity; (2) varied individual risk-reduction resources; (3) limited knowledge of any particular risk environment; and (4) fluctuating risk acceptability from person to person make a philosophical conception of how much risk persons should be exposed to next to impossible to develop. That risks known to be severe, highly probable, and easily fixable should be remediated is ethically obvious, but dilemmas over risk remediation never involve such scenarios. The more typical challenge, whether for the individual faced with a health risk or the health professional faced with limited resources and an always imperfect technological environment, is figuring out which risks are "reasonably" tolerable and which ones exceed those limits such that they should be eliminated. Further complicating matters is that risk anxieties and tolerances may vary for at least four "risk bearers": patients, treating clinicians, healthcare institutions, and insurers. The acceptability of risk can differ among them according to the following variables, which shape the character of vigilant practice.[21]

1. Availability of risk information. If, in the name of liberal values, a society decides to honor individual risk preference as much as possible but simultaneously wishes to exercise reasonable vigilance over extant risks, then accurate and comprehensible risk information must be available. Not only do individuals vary in their appetites for risk, but persons who cannot understand risks, or who choose not to understand them—such as those entering clinical trials thinking that the purpose of the trial is to benefit them or that they have nothing to lose—raise the question of how much risk insight and knowledge one needs before engaging in such risk taking. Furthermore, just determining the accuracy of risk information, even from data appearing in high-impact journals, can be daunting. On the other hand, sometimes risk information is known but not disclosed to the risk bearers, as in the following case:

Case 2.5. The patient, whom I'll call Amy, had been born with a neurologic condition called Wolf-Hirschhorn syndrome, a developmental disorder characterized by prenatal and postnatal growth impairment, pronounced intellectual disability, severe and delayed psychomotor development, seizures, and hypotonia, or poor muscle tone. At 13 years old, she weighed less than 40 pounds, did not speak, and could not walk independently. Amy had a complex medical history beginning at birth, and her pediatrician began to worry about new symptoms that suggested further musculoskeletal deterioration. He recommended that she receive home physical therapy, to which her parents agreed.

About a month into the therapy sessions, Amy's physical therapist positioned her in a squat position on the floor, with the therapist sitting behind her, gently rocking her back and forth with the aim of stretching Amy's hip muscles. As she did so, there was a loud "pop" from one of Amy's legs. The therapist immediately called 911, and x-rays confirmed a nasty spiral fracture of the femur.

In what would be an ill-advised move, the therapist discontinued all communications with the family, who were left feeling acutely distressed over what had happened. As they learned more about the nature of the therapy Amy had been receiving, they were further upset to learn that the ultimate goal had been to get her to sit upright unassisted, holding her head up for about 10 seconds. The exercises might have also relieved some of the contractures Amy had been developing, but that couldn't be assured.

Amy's parents decided to sue. They were especially upset that the therapist had never conducted an adequate informed consent discussion with them, in which she could have discussed the risks of a bone fracture as well as the projected benefits of the treatment. Although Amy's medical records attested to her fragile bone structure—which was also plainly visible for anyone to see—the therapist contended that such informed consent was not something she commonly did. Amy's parents countered, however, that had they known the goals of Amy's therapy—which they now considered inconsequential— they likely would not have consented to the therapy in the first place. Amy's lawyer further argued that the therapist was negligent either in being too aggressive with Amy's care program, such that the manipulation caused the fracture, or in failing to inform the parents of the therapy's risks, which materialized. (A veteran therapist with whom I discussed the case opined that the exercises Amy had been doing likely improved her muscle tone, which may have stressed her leg bones. In her opinion, the leg fracture was not all that unexpected, a foreseeable treatment risk that should have been conveyed to the parents.) Unfortunately, Amy's recovery from the leg fracture was lengthy and marked by clinical complications. The case settled out of court.

What struck me about the case, which happened more than two decades ago, was the therapist's surprise at the notion that she should incorporate informed consent into her physical therapy practice; she wanted to deny that physical therapy posed a significant enough risk of harm to her patients that needed to be communicated. Today, we would consider the failure of securing that informed consent an inarguable wrong precisely because we recognize the informational right of patients. Still, patients and research participants often have little idea of the risks they are assuming even after a comprehensive informed consent process.[22]

Even if factually accurate information is widely available, we face another, more philosophical problem: When have we reduced the denominator of risk *enough*? Is it enough to reduce a risk of, say, ventilator-acquired pneumonia to 1 in every 3,000 cases or 1 in every 5,000 cases? The ethically ideal number would be infinitesimally small but not zero, as that would be impossible. The reality—as opposed to the "ideality"—is the need to weigh the costs of achieving such reductions against the risk-reduction benefit itself. When are such reductions simply not worth it?

2. *Cost/benefit trade-offs.* Consider how many end-of-life interventions are last-chance therapies, or how many research trials have a very low probability of any kind of benefit. Yet, individuals will vary in their cost-benefit assessments. Andrea Phelps and her colleagues found, for instance, that persons of a deep Christian faith were more likely than non-Christians to opt for aggressive, life-prolonging treatments even in the face of poor survival odds or probability estimations, while Vyjeyanthi Periyakoil and her colleagues reported that physicians diagnosed with terminal conditions were much less likely than nonphysicians to opt for unpleasant but possibly life-prolonging treatments.[23,24] These examples speak to the subjectivity of risk assumption and how different people faced with the same levels of risk may vary in how they weigh their substantive cost/benefit probabilities. For example, consider in Case 2.2 the sexual violence enabled by architectural flaws in psychiatric units versus the estimated renovation costs to mitigate that risk. Now suppose that nothing bad has happened thus far, making the risk level seem acceptable and the decision to forgo physical improvements to the units reasonable. When a patient is sexually attacked, however, and a jury returns a million-dollar verdict in favor of the plaintiff, the cost of the prior decision to defer maintenance will seem unwise.

Situations like these pose the problem of optimism bias, which can cloud reasoning about safety issues, especially as an institution considers perhaps thousands of harm possibilities when deciding where to invest its resources. Healthcare environments are replete with harm opportunities, some likely common, while others might be quite unusual. For example, risk managers might be tasked with developing organizational policies on illegal substances discovered in a patient's possession; creating a response plan for staff members who are involved as "second victims" in serious, harm-causing medical error scenarios; formulating an error disclosure policy or a policy for an active shooter or a suicidal jumper on the premises; establishing a policy for a suspended physician who is re-entering practice;

devising training on how to chart medical errors and preventable adverse events; and creating a drug testing policy for all employees or a policy on placing transgender patients in semiprivate rooms. Some organizations might robustly undertake policy development in these areas, while others might devote their energies elsewhere—possibly not even undertaking a proactive risk-mitigation program because of resource constraints or organizational indifference. Of course, how an organization perceives the balance of risk frequency and magnitude will shape how it weighs these costs and benefits.

   3. *Balance of risk frequency and risk magnitude.* Risk management occurs amid an ongoing struggle between production pressures and human safety.[25] When any preventable harm materializes—whether low-frequency, high-harm events, like the BP oil disaster in the Gulf of Mexico, or high-frequency, low-harm occurrences, like most medication errors—it means that a harm pathway has been allowed to develop, exploiting human performance weaknesses, system design flaws, and knowledge imperfections.[6] Low-frequency, high-harm events lead to ignoring disaster possibilities because long stretches of nothing bad happening dull our risk awareness. When disasters ultimately occur, the natural urge is to blame, especially if the harmful event makes headlines. In contrast, high-frequency, low-harm occurrences often seem like business as usual, especially because they are usually remedied quickly and without much resource utilization.[26]

   Determining risk tolerance and mitigation will obviously require calculating the amount of effort required to reduce these risks, since a lot of effort devoted to preventing a low-frequency, low-magnitude risk seems imprudent, while a small amount of effort that would prevent a high-frequency, high-harm event is an organizational imperative. A key ethical problem in determining the acceptability of particular risks—because it involves prioritizing effort and making value-laden decisions—inheres in the details of those risks: some, like the architectural remodeling of units, may considerably stretch an organization's financial resources; other projects more amenable to organizational change may nevertheless require complex benefit-burden determinations, such as the decision to disclose any and all errors that reach a patient or to initiate a program of random drug testing for all employees.

   These kinds of initiatives not only reveal the moral conscience of an institution—since its financial and operational commitment to patient safety reflects the moral sensibilities of the institution's leadership—they also require a serious commitment to continuous patient safety learning. That knowledge acquisition never ends. The more hazards health professionals are exposed to and learn about in their environments, the more they are able to launch multiple responses that mitigate risk and harm.

4. *Baseline measures.* Baseline measures are indispensable in risk acceptability estimations because accurate information provides direction and content for risk awareness programs, management interventions, and evaluations of the success of risk-reduction efforts. Moreover, if a hospital or clinic is considering a particular expenditure to reduce a specific risk—say, the purchase of some new technology to reduce errors in pharmacy dispensing or in interpreting pathology specimens or radiologic images—the institution will want to compare the projected costs of such technology with the probability and the gravity of the relevant risk materialization. Such utilitarian-like calculations might sound cold, even ethically irresponsible, because they seem to translate people's welfare into numbers, but multiple goods are always in competition with one another such that benefit-burden trade-offs affecting patient care are utterly inevitable. Obviously, the accuracy of baseline measures informs the content of error wisdom and is critical to justifying patient safety decisions. The problem is that we often make decisions with inaccurate measures, whose imperfections we only learn about after harm has struck.

MacArthur "genius grant" recipient Peter Pronovost and his colleague Elizabeth Colantuoni commented on three strategies for managing the risk of harm per its preventability.[27] The first strategy is to assume, as do airlines, that all harm is preventable; the second is to use risk analytics to adjust for confounding variables like illness severity, patient demographics, and comorbid conditions and diagnoses; and the third correlates treatments to outcomes. Pronovost and Colantuoni abandon the first for reasons I've already discussed: healthcare providers have nowhere near the control of risk variables that airlines and similar organizations do. As such, expecting to prevent all harm is simply unreasonable (and even unwise for airlines if, for example, airfare costs would dramatically increase if airlines spent large amounts of money to eliminate a harm we might all be able to live with, such as baggage delays or losses). Second, adjusting harm-prevention efforts according to illness severity begs the question of illness severity's disconnection from the care process or how complications, the trauma of exposure to hospital care, and length of stay affect severity as well. Given the limited state of medical knowledge, we cannot perform these calculations with much confidence, because in so many cases, we don't know how harm prevention fluctuates with the nature and severity of a person's illness and all the variables that can affect it. (Plaintiff lawyers are faced with this problem constantly, as they must persuasively show that negligence more likely than not caused a patient's demise, which given a patient's ills may at best amount to speculation.)[28]

Pronovost and Colantuoni then proceed to agree with the idea I'm advancing on acceptable versus unacceptable risk of harm: "If the evidence-based therapy or standard was not rendered or was rendered incorrectly and the patient sustains the adverse outcome, the outcome would be labeled a preventable harm."[27(p1274)] In other words, if harm occurred by way of an unjustifiable deviation from the standard of care—assuming there is one—then that harm should be deemed preventable. No patient should be expected to endure that risk. Still, this nostrum ignores the myriad problems connected with nonobvious risk; for example, if Dr. Williams has a slightly higher postsurgical infection rate than Dr. Jones, how do we manage risk exposure for Dr. Williams's versus Dr. Jones's patients? Similarly, how do we manage risk exposure for patients requiring emergency room care over a holiday weekend, when adverse outcomes are known to increase?[29]

I suggest—and explore further in chapter 6—that the most disturbing question about ethics-based estimations of risk involves risk's unpredictably and obscurity. Even the presumably safest procedures carry risk, while palpably unsafe acts can sometimes cause no adversity, giving the illusion that the risk probability is low. Furthermore, as Richard Cook points out in his interview, we oftentimes come to appreciate risks post hoc, possibly because we resist imagining how harm might occur in a particular environment because such contemplation is too painful. So, we proceed with an "ignorance is bliss" mindset only to be shocked when disaster strikes. Training programs can teach vigilance (and mindfulness) skills, but healthcare professionals will need to proactively and continuously pursue such learning despite their organizations' productivity demands.

Conclusion: Vigilance and Its More Concrete Manifestations

As mentioned early in this chapter, vigilance implies—indeed, it originates and evolves from—a "knowing what and where to look" capacity that embodies highly contextualized knowledge of relevant hazards and risks. The delivery of a clinical intervention is always contextual, as its successful execution must respect its ecological details and accompanying risks. James

Reason has remarked that the difference between the expert and the amateur is that the expert has "a large stock of appropriate routines to deal with a wide variety of contingencies."[30(p18)] If true, then one cannot know enough about responding to hazards and risks, given the plethora of things that can go awry and occasionally surprise even the most veteran professional.

An experienced vigilance connotes the ability to fashion adaptive responses that mitigate or remove harm risks, that halt harm in the making, or that contain the severity of harm should it begin to materialize. Reason's observation on expertise is transdisciplinary. Retired master-sergeant Paul Howe, who served in special operations in high-risk encounters during his more than 20 years in the US Army, described the development of "a large stock of appropriate routines to deal with a wide variety of contingencies . . . Subconsciously, after years of training and combat, I learned 'where to look' and not waste valuable time scanning the entire area. Instead of looking at everything in the environment, walls, trees, cars, roofs, etc., I focused on where a person could shoot at you from. If you tried to look at everything, you are already getting behind in the loop because you are overloading your brain with useless information and images."[31(p8)]

Thus far, I have used the word "vigilance" to relate to an awareness of environmental or external harm threats, while in the chapters that follow, I use "mindfulness" as a more subjective, internally oriented posture of perception and attention that monitors one's own cognitive performance and its failures. I conclude this chapter, then, with some practical examples of what we can learn from vigilance failures gleaned from the various malpractice cases described in this chapter and in the previous one:

- *Comprehensive knowledge of how things can go wrong.* Vigilance must be informed, as illuminated especially in cases 2.1 (acetylcysteine overdose), 1.5 (ventilator disaster), and 2.4 (postsurgical blindness). A host of insensitivities to the possibility of things going wrong strongly suggests a lack of foresight among system operators, which can elevate patients' risk exposure to a system's weaknesses and vulnerabilities. The great irony, which history has taught us, is that an acute awareness of risk and danger usually requires the clinician to have witnessed or experienced their materialization firsthand.[1] Thus, organizations should create an atmosphere of transparency and anxious concern about such encounters and gather and disseminate this knowledge among staff, who shouldn't need to witness safety lapses directly to recognize their possibility.

- *Knowledge of the patient.* As reported in a study by Elizabeth Henneman and her colleagues, quintessential to a comprehensive knowledge of what could go wrong is "knowing the patient."[32] The authors note that this knowledge requires obtaining an accurate and inclusive report from a transferring unit or at change of shift; establishing relationships with the patient and his or her family; knowing the patient's response to past and present therapies; and reading his or her history. Note how these safety moments were missed in Case 2.1 (acetylcysteine overdose), in which the receiving unit and personnel at change of shift seemed disconnected from the previous shift; and how the sulfa allergy case (Case 1.1) suggested that the patient's care providers didn't acquaint themselves adequately with the patient's history.

- *Awareness of production pressures.* These demands loomed large in contributing to the outcomes in cases 2.2 (sexual violence in psychiatric units), 2.3 (retained laparotomy pad), and 2.4 (postsurgical blindness). The pressure to meet production targets compromises vigilance by tempting system operators to take shortcuts, make unjustifiably optimistic assumptions that increase risk, and believe that as long as no catastrophes have recently transpired, the system is reasonably safe. Yet, precisely in such moments, the point defining the classic safety-efficiency tension moves toward and perhaps crosses over the outer edge of the safety envelope.[28]

Although more a product of mindfulness than vigilance, *excessive optimism combined with assumption errors* is a natural response to production pressures that encourages taking shortcuts and other deviations from standards, rules, and policies. System operators who are expected to meet challenging production quotas will understandably compensate for their vigilance omissions by developing an unwarranted degree of confidence that everything will work well enough and that the performance of their fellow system operators will be reliable. Thus, overconfidence might especially occur where it should least occur: in recognized areas of weak system operations, for example, unreliable or chronically delayed interpretations of lab tests, inadequate bed availability on certain units, inadequately trained colleagues, or suboptimal care on holidays or off-peak shifts. Recall how in Case 2.1 (acetylcysteine overdose), nearly all personnel trusted the erroneous medication order and failed to follow the hospital's various policies for checking medication order accuracy.

- *Optimal physical environment, equipment upkeep, and documentation.* Cases 1.5 (ventilator disaster) and 2.2 (sexual violence in psychiatric units) vividly illustrate how degraded or suboptimal environments lay the groundwork for disasters. Yet, those lessons oftentimes sink in only after adversity strikes, and personnel wonder how they could have been so complacent about the system's safety. Likely, the unpleasantness of cultivating a "feral vigilance" as well as a staff that has never been sensitized to the possibilities of harm-causing error encourage a blasé attitudinal and normative posture toward risk. Poor, inaccurate, or unread documentation is apparent in cases 2.1 (acetylcysteine overdose) and 2.3 (retained laparotomy pad), while in Case 1.1 (sulfa allergy), multiple attestations to the patient's sulfa allergy were present in her medical records, but the attending physician and his staff missed or didn't read them.

- *Ongoing effective teamwork and communication.* Safety is a property of systems, and safer systems are those whose personnel have shared goals, clearly delineated roles, and mutual trust. The 2016 IOM report on diagnostic errors especially noted that "[n]urses need to be full and active members of the diagnostic team, with opportunities to present their observations and conclusions to other team members,"[33(p4.9)] recommending that nurses "be the eyes of the diagnostic team in detecting, reporting, and documenting changes in . . . [the] patient's symptoms, signs, complaints, or conditions."[33(p4.10)] Communication plays an indispensable role in these efforts by enabling personnel to gain consistent knowledge of the system's operations so that the adjustments and tweaks emphasized by Hollnagel and Reason can be made more successfully. Alternatively, when such communications fail—such as incomplete or inaccurate information at patient hand-offs or the failure to communicate lab results to the attending physician and staff— the likelihood of harm materialization increases. Also, the ultimate beneficiary of the system's operations—the client or patient—has a right to know about the system's anticipated deliverables and therefore should be included in certain of those communications. Thus, in Case 2.5 (physical therapy fracture risk), the decision makers' right to information highly relevant to their hopes and concerns was disappointed. Depriving patients of important information precludes their contribution to improving the system's safety. Again, if vigilance operates best amid the most comprehensive knowledge available, then not taking advantage of the collective knowledge of system personnel and patients seems shortsighted.

- *Involvement of patients and families.* Oddly, the imperfect knowledge base of healthcare safety is universally admitted, yet the idea of supplementing that knowledge with reports from the very individuals who have experienced harm-causing error is frequently forgone. Involving patients and families in maintaining safety remains a challenge for multiple reasons. Some patients will not speak up for fear of being labeled as complaining, difficult, neurotic, or stupid.[33(p4.14)] Professionals sometimes make snap judgments about patients, deciding after one look at a person that he or she will not be able to contribute anything significant to the diagnostic or treatment effort. On a more constructive note, the IOM report on diagnostic errors recommends that health professionals improve their communication skills. Organizations should commit themselves to pursuing educational programs that cultivate relational excellence among staff and their patients. Institutions might emphasize the importance of understanding health literacy; insist that professionals use "teach-back" techniques that improve patient understanding; and invite representatives from local patient populations whose native language or culture can compromise their communications and interactions with health professionals.[34] The IOM report also endorses patients having access to their medical records, an idea that some health professionals resist (just as they resist patient requests to audio record conversations), but in a society that increasingly insists on information to the point of overload, that sort of access seems inevitable.[33(p4.25)] The OpenNotes initiative, which allows patients to view the notes recorded by healthcare professionals during a clinical visit, was warmly received by patients involved in the OpenNotes study, in which 70 to 80 percent of respondents claimed they understood their care plans better and felt better prepared for clinical visits.[35] At the very least, considering that patients and their insurers have paid for those data, denying them access seems like a breach of contract. Concerns that patients may misinterpret their health information are easily countered by noting the opportunities patients have to correct their misunderstandings and the overall benefit of being at least somewhat informed when patients sit down with their physicians to discuss their symptoms.

H. G. Wells's observation that "[c]ivilization is a race between education and catastrophe" applies superbly well to healthcare environments and to our daily confrontation with life's inherent risks.[36] The vigilant person is one who suspects or knows where harm opportunities reside and how their materialization might be contained or eliminated. This implies, however, that the sentinels of risk—patient safety, risk-management, and quality-improvement personnel—will relentlessly study, disseminate information, perform continuous review, and train their staffs. Vigilance entails risk awareness as well as educated risk tolerance. And while error may seem intolerable, like risk it is inevitable. In the next chapter, I survey some of error's attributes through the second of our analytic lenses: mindfulness.

Interview with Richard Cook

Richard Cook is a research scientist in the Department of Integrated Systems Engineering and a clinical professor of anesthesiology at the Ohio State University (OSU) in Columbus. Dr. Cook is an internationally recognized expert on patient safety, medical accidents, complex system failures, and human performance at the sharp end of these systems. He has investigated various problems in such diverse areas as urban mass transportation, semiconductor manufacturing, military software, and internet-based business systems. He is often a consultant for not-for-profit organizations, government agencies, and academic groups. His most often cited publications are "Gaps in the Continuity of Patient Care and Progress in Patient Safety," "Operating at the Sharp End: The Complexity of Human Error," "Adapting to New Technology in the Operating Room," *A Tale of Two Stories: Contrasting Views of Patient Safety*, and "Going Solid: A Model of System Dynamics and Consequences for Patient Safety." Dr. Cook graduated with honors from Lawrence University, where he was a Scholar of the University. He worked for Control Data Corporation in supercomputer systems design and engineering applications before earning his MD degree from the University of Cincinnati in 1986. From 1987 until 1991, he did research on expert human performance, safety, and human error at OSU. He completed an anesthesiology residency at OSU in 1994 and is ABA board certified. From November 1994 until March 2012, he was a practicing anesthesiologist, teacher, and researcher in the Department of Anesthesia and Intensive Care at the University of Chicago. He was professor of healthcare systems safety at Kungliga Tekniska Högskolan, Sweden's Royal Institute of Technology, from April 2012 through June 2015, and is now professor emeritus of the same field. In September 2015, he returned to work at OSU.

JB: Richard, I'm delighted to have your thoughts in my book because you were the person who, over 20 years ago, turned me on to error and its related literature. I can never thank you enough for the inspiration and the provocative work you've done on it. So, I'd like to start with your giving me an overview of your thoughts on error and risk as they've developed or changed over your career.

RC: Well, my experience with this spans over 30 years. I've seen things come and go, and I've seen cycles of thinking and different approaches and ideas around patient safety arrive and depart. The impression I get is that patient safety remains a difficult area for organizations. What we are seeing now reflects more a continuing struggle than any resolution. Much of the territory remains conflicted and controversial. Some people tried to bring an end to what they see as dilatory, somewhat academic efforts to understand the deeper problems. These problems arise at the juncture of forces in healthcare that are frankly incompatible; yet working through those incompatibilities moment by moment, daily, weekly, or monthly is what safety is all about.

Safety should not be thought of as a noun but as a verb. People try to work out acceptable solutions in ways that are compatible with all the pressures they face. In the modern world, people are able to manage those pressures fairly successfully most of the time. Most of the time, things work pretty well. The only time we look closely at our systems is when they are not going well—no one calls me at three o'clock in the morning to tell me that everything is going fine. Then we are struck by those conflicting demands and pressures. What we call "error" is really our conclusion that the people involved have judged poorly how to navigate those conflicting pressures. We ignore the fact that those conflicts are inevitable and enduring, and they change in unpredictable ways that seldom get attention.

JB: So talk about the conflicts and incompatibilities that you just referred to.

RC: The most obvious one, described by Erik Hollnagel, is the efficiency-thoroughness trade-off. This is trade-off space. We are always being confronted with the need to look more closely, take more time, be more deliberate, and, simultaneously, to search out more efficient ways of getting things done. But there are no absolute criteria to locate where we should be in that trade-off space, and we are constantly moving around in that trade-off space. This is necessarily so. The world is structured sometimes nicely and sometimes not nicely, and sometimes in ways that we can move quickly and take advantage of things, and sometimes in ways where it's not prudent to do so. And you can see this in your everyday world: the way you drive, the way you make your coffee, the way you make your lists of things to do—virtually everything you do indicates the ways you negotiate this trade-off space between being efficient and being thorough. This also applies macroscopically to organizations in terms of production and performance.

JB: And in medicine you're always dealing with uncertainty.

RC: There's an inherent uncertainty in patients; they are different from one another. Our ability to understand these differences and their implications is quite limited. For example, while we have plenty of guidelines for treating disease X or disease Y, we rarely see anyone with just disease X or disease Y. For me to see a patient who isn't taking at least three medications is very unusual.

There's an old saying in surgery: "If there are more than two operations for any condition, none of them are any good." And that's a really telling observation, because if we have something that works well, we use it. The other one that you'll remember from your childhood is that if you're going to be in a fight, don't throw your second-best punch first. So we never choose to use the lesser quality thing when the better one is well established and understood. The problem is we're often not choosing according to primary or main effects but according to side effects, between tolerability and other consequences. So if you're taking a statin for hypercholesterolemia, the likelihood is that you may develop leg cramps; and in some severe cases, you could develop rhabdomyolysis, which can cause your muscles or your kidneys to break down; or you might go on to develop diabetes.

What we think of as error is really a post facto evaluation of performances that had outcomes that we don't like. We are trapped by our strong belief that the circumstances before the outcome were obviously indicating that we should do *x* and not *y*. But this is an artifact of hindsight bias.

What I've described just now is a scientific view of "error" that's been well empirically verified over the years. However, that view has run up against organizational and institutional imperatives that require being essentially reassured that things are OK. To be in an environment of uncertainty is politically unacceptable. The organization keeps insisting that it is safe because this is an image that must be maintained if the organization is to remain intact and the leadership to retain authority. This is a primary reason that "human error" continues to be so popular.[37] So, they treat bad outcomes as problems to be solved, not information about how the world works.

A central problem with patient safety is that medical people are so facile with language. They are exceptionally skilled at appearing to embrace ideas and themes without understanding them in a deep way. I think this has been true for both the quality and safety movements, both of which were largely neutered by their contact with medical practice. Both safety and quality were originally unreachable ideals, the pursuit of which would [create] a much better world. The incessant pursuit of quality and safety, although demonstrably incomplete and unsuccessful, would engender a purposeful transformation of work and organization. (That's [W. Edwards] Deming in a nutshell.) But if you look at the quality world in medicine, rather than quality being an unreachable ceiling, it has become a very reachable floor—that is, a level below which performance shall not fall. While giving eloquent lip service to Deming and the great safety thinkers, in many places, safety today is mostly a mélange of metric madness and organizational fantasies about best practice. The rationale is simple: as long as the indicators tell us we're above a particular floor, then we can do whatever we want with our system. We can increase demands for production, we can cut costs, we can reduce this, we can reduce that, and so long as our indicators tell us we haven't fallen below this floor, we have safety.

JB: Do you think that's unreasonable, though, setting that bottom-line floor?

RC: It depends on what counts as reasonable. The consequences of willful ignorance are severe. Medicine and surgery are taking place in a dynamic world, where everything is changing all the time. Indeed, the rate of change is exceptionally high, especially in our field. So past performance doesn't tell us very much about what performance will be in the future. The patient safety movement started because of events that reflected deep and previously unappreciated vulnerabilities in our system. Recall the 1995 Ben Kolb case from Martin Memorial Hospital.[38] This tragedy seemed to come out of the blue. It did not just surprise—it astonished. This was not something anticipated, counted up over time, or added to a collection, but a kind of sui generis event. The world of medicine and surgery continues to produce these kinds of events at a fairly high rate. The problem with performance as a floor is that it is necessarily insensitive to these things; it cannot and does not appreciate them.

We continue to embrace the "those responsible have been sacked" approach to safety. This allows us to divide the outcomes we like from those we do not. The desirable outcomes we assign to "the system." The undesirable ones we chalk up to human frailty. So the system is either safe and efficient, or its faults are due to human failures, which can be penalized. That's the best of all possible worlds for the people running the system. Heads I win, tails you lose.

JB: Let's get back to the Ben Kolb case, though, because it demonstrates something that I want to talk about in my book, which is foreseeability. What happened there should have been foreseeable: We should have realized that sooner or later, someone was going to mix up the epinephrine with the lidocaine. So, am I on the right track with my emphasizing a lack of foreseeability, or is the view that you're giving me going in a different direction?

RC: The notion of foreseeability is heavily bound to hindsight. An event's occurrence makes it seem more likely in hindsight than it did in foresight. This is a function of our cognitive processes as post facto reviewers. The world is filled with hazards. Of the many hazards that are present in the world, this one turns out to be important, and the actor should have foreseen it then because it is obvious to us now. Frankly, I don't buy that at all. In fact, I think it's a misstatement of what's happening. One problem with events like Ben Kolb's death is that they are like flashbulb memories. They create a misleading appearance of crispness that is an artifact of the event's *magnitude*. It doesn't reflect the way the event transpired. The people in the room at the time not only didn't foresee that, they didn't believe it possible. It was only the phenomenally determined investigation of the event by Doni Haas that led to the conclusion that exchanging epinephrine for lidocaine was the mechanism. No one at the time knew what was going on. So, I don't buy the foreseeability argument. I think that what happens is we assume that the hindsight bias doesn't exist, such that what was foreseeable in retrospect should have been foreseeable prospectively. The problem, though, is not with people's foreseeing; it's a problem with our retrospective hindsight bias.

JB: So it sounds to me like what you're putting forward here is quite different from what someone like James Reason puts forward in terms of cognitive traps. Where he seems to emphasize perception and cognition, you seem to emphasize the environment's demands on the system operator.

RC: I don't think there's a big incompatibility between my view and Reason's. I'm now focused on the organizational and consequential aspects of this, the postevent understandings and reactions rather than the pre-event sequences. And I'm trying to indict the postevent understandings because I think they are deeply flawed. The customary way of doing things is that they go well. When they don't, we point to a person or group as responsible.

In our monograph *A Tale of Two Stories: Contrasting Views of Patient Safety*, we pointed out that if you take as your starting point for understanding safety the investigation of when things go wrong, you are inevitably going to be biased in ways that will make that investigation inaccurate.[39] What you have to look for instead is why things *normally* go right, and why the activities, judgments, and decisions that usually make things work well in certain circumstances fail to make them work in others. Ultimately, we learn that the world is more variable, heterogeneous, and, yes, perverse than we had previously appreciated. Rather than looking at failures, we do better to look more closely for what the ordinary world has in it that creates performance successes and how people resolve their performance challenges.

JB: So does this recall in any way James Reason's swiss cheese model, where the holes have to line up just so in order for a disaster to go down?

RC: Yes, but in my view Reason was pursuing a kind of static or quasi-static world. We work in a dramatically and unpredictably changing world, and asking people to deal with that world without incurring any of the side effects or consequences of that newness—it grows harder to do that, especially as change accelerates. The present-day example of all this in medicine is the electronic medical record and all the problems that arise from dealing with this huge amount of data one screen at a time. It's like you have this little keyhole perspective on the data as you move from page to page. In fact, I wrote the dissent to the IOM report on medical records, where I contended that they were dangerous and were going to kill people. I think the last few years have somewhat vindicated my position.

JB: I must say I rarely hear physicians saying anything positive about them. Some, like Gordon Schiff, have been more optimistic, saying that the future of medical records can witness considerable improvement over what we have today, but it's pretty clear that we're going through a bad patch right now, at least according to the records users. Of course, we don't know how that future will turn out.

RC: The great science-fiction writer William Gibson wrote a short story called "The Gernsback Continuum," wherein he holds up the world imagined by the science-fiction writers of the 1930s and compares it to the reality of the 1980s. He basically said, here's the world they were imagining in the thirties, and here's how it turned out 50 years later; there is basically no similarity or relationship. And I think this is the problem of people who engage in techno fantasies: that the promises of technology seem to be unlimited, but the actual trajectory of change undermines the capital F future. I find it surprising that people continue to be surprised by the unpredictability of that trajectory.

JB: I want to get back to the metrics that you were talking about earlier, and I want to challenge you with something like, "Look, Richard, if we lower the rate of falls; if we lower the rate of ventilator-acquired pneumonias; if we lower our medication error rates, that's a good thing, isn't it?"

RC: Absolutely, and I believe in Mom and apple pie, too, but posing the question that way is somewhat prejudicial. You believe that the incidence of falls and infections are quasi-static events existing in a kind of repeatable, elemental, atomic environment; that there's such a thing as a "fall" that can be nicely encapsulated and measured. But remember, our systems don't keep track of "falls"; they keep track of "reports" of falls. And typically less than 5 percent of such events get reported, and the ones that get reported are usually the ones that are going to be discovered anyway from other events. So reporting is basically a defensive measure. Consequently, what does it mean to have metrics based on only 5 percent of the bad things that happen? Very often, such as in central line studies, they use a pretty weak definition of central lines that conjures up a placid background (rather than the very volatile one that really happens) and that can allow the incessant production pressure to continue.

The social and organization function of this story is not so much to say, "We are safe," as it is to say, "We are in control." The managers, administrators, the boards, and the organization owners need constantly to say they are managing these events in a competent fashion, that they are competent to run the show. And this is why every major event that becomes public is followed by some member of the senior administrative staff standing up and saying, "We're going to take action on this so that this can never happen again." That's nonsense. The statement relies on an understanding that's not even close to being complete, let alone true. But the statement is an element of a much larger purposeful construction: to create a bland and manageable image of safety that allows these production [pressures] to continue and authority to remain in place.

JB: So, in your view, would it be correct to say that a kind of "propaganda" has been created around patient safety?

RC: That would be putting the kindest construction on it. A more realistic construction is that the incessant economic pressure to make the system more efficient and reduce costs has led to people saying something like, "We recognize that all the things we initially understood as quality are not going to be achievable, so we'll replace them with these metrics that will be used as our substitute for quality or safety." In addition these metrics serve the purpose of wresting control of quality from a professional medical cadre and turning it over to an administrative/bureaucratic one. One of the great advantages of metrics is that they do not require interpretation. They can be compiled, evaluated, and disseminated by people who are not professionals. So what this whole safety metric does is to wrest control from a physician class—which is seen as self-interested and empowered—and give it to a bureaucratic class that is presumably objective and can make decisions based on good data. That's the transition that has occurred: the goal is to de-professionalize, in an assessment sense, what it means to be in control of the system.

JB: So, if you were king of patient safety, what would you like to see? What kinds of models or platforms would you prefer?

RC: I don't believe in the "king of the world" approach or a command-and-control economy. Huge top-down management systems work very poorly in rapidly changing environments. I believe that the bottom line is giving people on the front lines more authority to act independently. What we understand requires empowering people at the sharp edge, the front lines, by giving them the power and authority to undertake these things rather than locating that authority elsewhere.

JB: So where do standards and rules and regulations fit in?

RC: There's a paradox there because there is no "standard" standard of care. Standard of care is a moving target concocted out of a series of microscopic views of specific things, along with lots of inferences as to what those things mean. The assumption that it's possible to acquire and assemble large amounts of data that will somehow tell us what sorts of actions should occur at some future time is flat out wrong. That's the assumption of so-called evidence-based medicine: that by assembling large collections of data from a variety of different sources we can define what is best practice. Practically speaking, that doesn't work very well. A third of these evidence-based practices are invalid by the time they appear; another third are so obscure that it's hard to know how to apply them; the rest are interesting, but there are so many variables at play that figuring out where they apply is quite hard.

JB: And there are all those comorbidities to contend with that destabilize predictive power.

RC: Precisely. And the other thing I don't like about them is that they say, "Here's what you need to do, but there may be clinical circumstances that require you to do something else. And by the way, then you should do whatever else there is that you need to do." It means, "You should do what I tell you to unless you shouldn't do what I tell you, but you should nevertheless be able to tell what the situation requires." And because of the hindsight bias, if you didn't use the care path, and things turned out poorly, then people will ask why you didn't; and if you did use the "standard," and things didn't turn out well, they'll say that this was a special case, so why didn't you depart from the standard?"

Standards aren't so much guides for performance as they are means of making assessments of performance, especially after performances we don't like. They are designed to allow us to do this in a way that gives the appearance of evenhandedness. We want some sort of external rule that can be used as a guide for how to behave. But the issue is always, How do you interpret these things? The goal is to be able to have extrinsic standards for evaluation and to call them concrete or objective. But it's not about performance; it's about evaluations of performance.

JB: So in the language of ethics, you would be called a fine-grained particularist. That is, you tend to see situations as radically unique, as affected by a tremendous number of variables that make them so, and therefore that we would have to place a premium on the judgment of the system operator. There's a real parallel with ethical decision making and learning. Just as with standards of care in medicine, you're supposed to know what standard applies and then know how to apply it; in ethics, you're supposed to know which principle—so think of autonomy, nonmaleficence, beneficence, and justice—applies and how to apply in a given case.

RC: I would also say that principles don't speak for themselves. The act of applying them is the ethical act.

JB: So, Richard, we've been talking about an hour, and you've been enormously kind, but I want to ask you what do you see over the next 5, 10, 20 years of patient safety? Do you see more of the same? Do you expect to be disappointed, or do you think there might be some really positive changes? And what kind of changes would you like to see?

RC: As I said at the beginning, I think the conflicts are inexorable, and they are derived from the world around us. As long as we treat safety as something atomic, as separated from those things, we'll always be frustrated, because the conflicts will be hidden. It is therefore productive to point out how safety is the working out of what to do in the face of the ordinary, frustrating, misbehaved world. The greatest challenge we now face is the one we haven't discussed: that we have built a system in which it has become increasingly harder for people to realize that they are faced with ethical challenges and that they must cope with them. The thing I am most concerned about is that the social contract that used to be an implicit part of medical practice—that we're going to give you a large piece of authority but also a great deal of responsibility to carry—is no longer clear, and that this discourages people from understanding that they are in human relationships with patients, that they are in a relationship that requires questioning. The deprofessionalization of medicine and surgery has had the effect of making people—on both sides of the scalpel—instrumental rather than human. Our goal should be to fight against that tide.

I ask every resident I work with to find out the patient's occupation. In the timeout before surgery, I try to explain to everyone in the room who this person *is*. We'll find out things like, the person we're going to operate on is taking care of two small children who are her daughter's because her daughter is presently incarcerated. Or that the man we're going to operate on is a retired police officer who now spends his time teaching children how to play chess. Or that this frail elderly man once fought at Bastogne. In every case, it seems to me that the way we make progress is to return to patients the quality of being unique, irreplaceable human beings. And that that is the single most important thing we can do. If I were to change anything about this, it would be to recognize patients as human beings rather than as bodies with an illness. Because I think everything flows from that—everything about what it means to act ethically flows from *I-thou* and not from *I-it*.

JB: And as you say, it is the inexorability of medicine's reductionistic sensibility that removes us from that humanness. The possibility of replacing humans with machines; the reduction of humans not just to cells and molecules but to Higgs boson particles.

RC: This is the danger, of course, but I am optimistic. Physicians, surgeons, nurses, pharmacists, and therapists are our greatest resource for overcoming this trend. They have regular, close contact with real human suffering, fear, and anguish. They appreciate the great power they have by virtue of their knowledge, expertise, and position. They understand that with this great power comes great responsibility.

JB: It gets us back to those QA [quality assurance] measures you were talking about: that administration has something they can talk about in an atomistic, measurable way that allows them to make a more persuasive case for the cases they want to make.

RC: Maybe you should get those people to read this book.

JB: Richard, as always, my thanks.

RC: You're welcome.

3   Mindfulness

We are ever vulnerable to seeing correlation as causation, misinterpreting things simply because of temporal relationships, suckered by logical fallacies, seeing meaningful patterns where none exist, and are completely fooled by illusions and magicians.

Pat Croskerry[1(p23)]

Question: What's the most commonly missed fracture in the emergency room?
Answer: The second one.

Karen Lommel on Twitter[2]

Chapter Overview: This chapter focuses on medical epistemology, that is, on the thinking processes of clinicians as they ponder the symptom presentations of their patients. Topics in the first part include a discussion of human-thinking imperfections as illustrated by the phenomenon of diagnostic error. Diagnosis is especially highlighted because it may well represent the prototypical medical manifestation of thinking, decision making, and analysis, and because it has witnessed considerable research over the last decade on how diagnostic error occurs. Embedded in all this is a discussion of *medical metacognition,* or thinking about thinking in medicine. In the second part, I examine the nature of *medical mindfulness* and associated strategies for achieving it, again as especially relevant to diagnostic errors. The chapter concludes with a listing of mindfulness strategies (see box 3.1), discussion of the importance of feedback in the learning process, and an interview with Pat Croskerry, probably the premier international researcher on mindfulness in healthcare decision making.

PART I: DIAGNOSTIC ERROR AND CLINICAL REASONING

When patients visit their physicians, they have an inarguable right to expect their doctors to treat them according to the standard of care, or at least according to a standard of reasonableness. Clinicians' licenses are predicated on their reliably demonstrating proficiency and knowledge that, in the opinion of professionals authorized by a state, are sufficient for them to be allowed to practice medicine there. That proficiency is nicely captured by the demonstrated ability to treat patients according to what ordinary, reasonable, prudent physicians, nurses, or therapists would do in like or similar circumstances.[3]

Notice the gap, however, between possessing clinical knowledge as conveyed in classroom lectures, continuing medical education programs, learned texts, and peer-reviewed journal articles and treating patients according to what "ordinary, reasonable, prudent physicians, nurses, or therapists would do in like or similar circumstances." Obviously, the latter demonstration may not bear much similarity to the former. On the one hand, the "community" standard that defines "ordinary and reasonable" in a given geographic area—that is, what clinicians in that locality typically do—may be frankly Neanderthal or impossible to verify.[4] On the other hand, to expect all clinicians, regardless of how good willed and competent they seem, to have adequate knowledge about what to do in every clinical situation they encounter is unrealistic. Some futurists believe that within a few years, we will be able to access the entire PubMed database on treating a patient's complaints and symptoms and then be able to interrogate that information for a treatment plan (that takes into account the patient's lab findings and DNA).[5] Still, a clinician will have to decide whether to follow what the technology advises or do something else.[6]

But that day of advanced artificial intelligence (AI) may be a long way off. For now, I wish to pursue the ethical question of what Dr. Smith "owes" her patients epistemically and ethically when she enters the treatment room, introduces herself, and begins gathering treatment information. This chapter explores two responses. The first bears on the kinds of epistemic error traps, cognitive pitfalls, and knowledge gaps that will challenge Dr. Smith as she proceeds. Even assuming that Dr. Smith is feeling reasonably well that day and is not unduly distracted, disoriented, interrupted, or bothered, what kinds of cognitive challenges does she nevertheless face minute by minute that might compromise her "mindfulness" and precipitate error? Mark Graber's observation, "Medical diagnosis is essentially a special case of decision-making under conditions of uncertainty," is what primarily confronts Dr. Smith here, in the context of what Pat Croskerry has observed, that "medicine has put more emphasis on content knowledge than on how we think."[7(p553),1(p26)]

The second response is more substantive: How can we improve clinical decision making and medical reasoning? If error implicates only human beings because machines "malfunction" rather than "err," then what can be done to reduce the epistemic fallibility of healthcare professionals such that patients will receive treatments that result from intelligent medical reasoning informed by accepted and recognized standards of care?

This chapter is inspired by the concept and practice of *mindfulness*. Rimma Teper and her colleagues characterized mindfulness as comprising two facets: in-the-moment awareness combined with nonjudgmental acceptance of emotions and thoughts.[8] They and other mindfulness scholars stress that their notion of clinical mindfulness does not involve emptying the mind of thoughts and emotions, as some varieties of Eastern meditation encourage, but rather "increases sensitivity to affective cures in the experiential field" that can either compromise or enhance decision making.[8(p44),9] The hope is that mindfulness techniques and performance will alert professionals to when intrusive and unhelpful feelings are interfering with the practice of sound reasoning so that they can recruit their "regulatory" resources to improve cognitive accuracy and reliability. The goal, then, is to discipline attention and thinking in ways that attend to important rather than unimportant sensory inputs.

But the task is not an easy one. Slipping into careless thinking and feeling patterns is human nature, and mindfulness can require a lifetime of effort to maintain. The work is nevertheless well worth doing.

Clinical Ignorance, Cognitive Imperfections, and Diagnostic Error

Consider what it is like to be Dr. Smith as she begins listening to and probing her patient's complaints. The IOM's 2015 committee on diagnostic error proposed that physicians like her will typically engage in an *information-gathering* process that includes taking a clinical history, performing a physical exam, perhaps ordering diagnostic tests, and possibly referring the patient to a specialist or getting a consultation from another doctor.[9] Throughout this process, Dr. Smith is *integrating* the information she is gathering with additional data points acquired from lab results, family reports, and the patient's clinical history into a comprehensive interpretation of the patient's condition—in other words, a *diagnosis*, or an identification of the patient's disease or ailment. Ultimately, she communicates her presumptive diagnosis to the patient and perhaps to his or her family and then recommends a treatment plan. The treatment plan ensues, perhaps with follow-up visits, and the outcome is evaluated according to whatever success or failure criteria are in play.

My first area of interest is to examine the cognitive challenges that Dr. Smith or any physician confronts in collecting data, making a diagnosis, and developing a treatment plan. One particular insight is fundamental to this examination: Although some *diagnostic* errors will be attributable to system or processing errors (such as a lost mammogram or a failed communication), most will at least implicate cognitional, thinking, or sensory-processing errors.[10] Consider, then, the following types of errors, especially as they involve the diagnostic process:

- Diagnostic errors are probably the most common cause of medical malpractice litigation in the United States.[11] A prominent reason for the serious harm that diagnostic error can wreak is that a diagnostic mistake *early* in treating a patient can remain with that patient and enable subsequent mistakes downstream, such as in ordering unnecessary tests, calling in specialists who likewise don't pick up on the error, or prescribing treatments that are all predicated on the error.[12] Of course, a physician might also miss the diagnosis completely and allow the patient to walk out of the clinic without the kind of timely and appropriate treatment his or her condition requires. When the correct diagnosis is finally made, curative treatments might be unavailable.

- In a 2013 study by Hardeep Singh and colleagues on types of errors in primary care, physicians failed to document a differential diagnosis— that is, what else might account for the patient's complaints or symptoms—in 81.1 percent of cases.[13] Diagnostic errors often begin with the failure to consider likely diagnostic alternatives, perhaps suggesting a physician's overconfidence or his or her feeling rushed and needing to get through. Thus, when diagnostic errors that lead to significant harm are evident or are "more likely than not," defendants in malpractice trials will often find defending these errors difficult, and they will settle quickly.

- Faulty information synthesis, which may well be the most common source of diagnostic error, covers a wide range of factors, such as failing to discern an important symptom or sign, drawing an incorrect conclusion from the symptoms, not noticing that reported symptoms are unsubstantiated by observation or laboratory results, failing to appreciate and factor in aspects of the patient's situation relevant to the diagnosis, or ordering an inappropriate test to confirm a diagnosis.[9,14(p1496)] As suggested in the previous bullet point, its most common treatment manifestation may well be *premature closure*, which is the tendency to stop considering other possibilities after confidently reaching a hypothesis about what's causing the patient's symptoms.[14(p1497)]

- In Singh's 2013 primary care study, the most common information synthesis errors involved medical history taking (56.3 percent of errors), the physical examination (47.4 percent), diagnostic tests ordered for further workup (57.4), and the failure to review previous documentation (15.3 percent).[13] These findings are remarkable because they implicated diagnoses that were not occult or exotic but rather clinical conditions that any reasonably trained physician should have detected. If so, many physicians may need remediation on some of the more basic skills of the art of medicine and on those process or technological variables that can disturb what would normally be acceptable medical reasoning and judgment, such as the various cognitive traps described in this chapter.[15]

- A reliance on pattern or prototype recognition may also precipitate error, especially from premature closure.[14] For example, Dr. Smith may be so familiar with the patient's symptom presentation that she sees utterly no reason to search for an alternative explanation. *And usually, she will be right and commit no error.* Yet, she might also develop what the literature has called "clinical inertia," which is a "form of emotional resistance to changing long-held beliefs and attitudes . . . Many solutions and beliefs are well-established old friends that have given the clinician comfort in the past."[15(p350)] These old "cognitive friends" are the navigational tools a physician uses because they have proved themselves immensely reliable over time. Unfortunately, this sets up the clinician for error when a particular patient confounds his or her usually reliable epistemic source. So, if that occurs, Dr. Smith will need to have the cognitive skill set to recalibrate her bearings and consider a change. That, in turn, may suggest a revised judgment, which, one hopes, Dr. Smith will have the will and know-how to perform. Yet, she may resist the effort: "Practitioners find it difficult or impossible to know when additional information is worth the cost."[15(p35),2]

- How patients present their primary complaints and symptoms to physicians is a common cause of error, whereby such a presentation might divert the physicians' attention to unimportant, irrelevant, or secondary issues rather than to what standard diagnostic approaches would typically require.[16] Possibly, these physicians are too susceptible to an *anchoring* bias, wherein they are particularly attracted to and *cannot divert their attention from* a particular feature of the patient's symptom presentation, causing them to fail to attend to other, just as important items. Of course, patients may also be poor communicators, have low health literacy, be intimidated by or scared of the physician, and not be well positioned overall to collaborate with doctors on arriving at a diagnosis and an associated care plan.[17]

- Should one of Dr. Smith's patients experience a serious diagnostic mishap, as in Dr. Smith's failing to detect a malignancy, an analysis of the patient's misfortune will very likely show multiple contributing factors, virtually always involving system-related issues like poor communication, poor documentation, or delays in processing lab tests (or losing them).[18] Consequently, while cognitive errors are extremely common, clinical disasters usually involve faulty cognition combined with a faulty (social and/or technological) system. A 2009 study by Gordon Schiff and his colleagues of 538 physician-reported errors found that the most commonly missed diagnosis involved cancer, and the most common reasons that the cancer was misdiagnosed were faulty laboratory and radiologic testing (accounting for 44 percent of the errors) and erroneous clinical assessments (32 percent).[19] The latter especially included flawed hypothesis generation, mistakes in weighing or prioritizing findings, and failure to recognize urgency or complications.

- A 2009 study on radiology errors by Kshitij Mankad and colleagues found that although radiology errors are extremely common and figure prominently in medical malpractice suits, few of the radiologists studied kept any form of personal error record, and many did not attend error meetings.[20]

- Graber and coauthors reported in 2012 that radiologists in the United Kingdom must review 5,000 mammograms a year for certification, as opposed to 480 in the United States.[7] They also noted that the typical continuing medical education courses that US physicians attend throughout the year "generally have not led to substantial improvement in measured performance," although a highly focused, disease-specific training activity, such as improving recognition of subarachnoid hemorrhage, has shown some learning improvement.[7(p547)]

- *Bayesian diagnostic reasoning*, consisting of densely analytical, differential, probabilistic, inductive, and deductive data and algorithmic-driven processes that computer technologies perform, is exactly *unlike* what most seasoned physicians or nurses do on units. There they rely on pattern-recognition learning and memories encoded over decades, which serve them spectacularly well in the majority of their diagnostic encounters.[9(pp2.27-2.30)] But the health professional who overly relies on his or her experience will inevitably miss important factors, which can easily invite harm-causing misses.[21] The challenge presented to Dr. Smith requires her to insightfully know when she needs to dig deeper into the patient's history, symptoms, or laboratory findings, and when such digging amounts to a waste of time and medical resources.

Robert Wears and Christopher Nemeth have observed something that nicely captures a central message of these bullet points: "Rather than being misdiagnosed, the problem is misperceived, which explains why those who are later described as 'making the wrong diagnosis' saw it at the time as the only reasonable one to make."[21(p206)] Much of the literature on diagnostic error bears this out, such as how production pressures compress a physician's attention and decision making in ways that accommodate his or her anxious need to move on to the next patient; how pattern recognition, especially as it is learned and confirmed over time, will often result in dismissing contending diagnostic hypotheses or reasonable differential diagnoses as a waste of time; how knowledge limitations by their very nature reduce the scope of diagnostic or clinical options, imaginings, or reasonings, including the ways in which they can be corrupted by factors like availability and anchoring biases; and, of course, how a physician may be fatigued, sleep deprived, or cognitively overwhelmed with incoming information.[22] Also, whether physicians like or dislike a patient can affect their willingness to pay attention or ask an additional, sometimes remarkably valuable question like "Is there anything else you'd like to tell me?"

If the research on cognitive performance is correct, then whatever is coursing through Dr. Smith's neural circuits during any patient encounter is colored by her feeling that she is nearly always performing at an adequate if not superior skill level, and that she does not need to step back and critically review her thinking and reasoning.[23(pp41-49)] She doesn't do this because the effort strikes her as energy depleting and unnecessary.[24] Nevertheless, her unique epistemic challenges are exacerbated by her working in "a health care system in which test results are not easily tracked, patients are sometimes poor informants, multiple handoffs exist, and information gaps are the norm. For even the most stellar practitioners, clinical processes and judgments are bound to fail occasionally under such circumstances."[25(p494)] Even so, that system will generate many more successes than failures, and we must be grateful to Dr. Smith and her peers for stepping into that chaotic fray, caring for their patients, and splendidly succeeding with the majority. The great question is whether patient safety will improve over the coming decades, at least as long as it relies on the performance of human operators, who will always err, until error-prevention technologies using AI systems come along. Although I expect a great deal of progress, there will be plenty of lumps and bumps along the way, such as those discussed below.

Thinking about Thinking

One of the most prominent scholars in the field of diagnostic errors, Pat Croskerry, has noted that the elements of carefully examining how we think, that is, thinking about thinking, or *metacognition*, would include being aware of what is required to learn something; recognizing memory limitations; appreciating that data gathering is often *perspectival*—shaped and processed by an individual's unique cognitive and emotional equipment, psychohistory, values, training, and genetic makeup; having the capacity to self-critique performance and identify deficits and technical areas for improvement; and identifying and incorporating better cognitive approaches, and then self-monitoring them to determine if improvement actually occurs.[26] Ironically, this is why the hypothetical Dr. Smith rarely questions her knowledge gathering and synthesis: doing so would be strenuous, and to the extent that she suffers no negative feedback, she believes she is doing just fine. Yet, learning and practicing the metacognitive strategies Croskerry lists are priceless because they enable "stepping back from the pushes and pulls of the immediate situation" and displacing system operators from inside to outside themselves to better discern their flaws.[26(p118)] Simply urging people to be more careful or leaving them up to their own devices to improve usually doesn't work. Although many people would grant that other perspectives on or interpretations of "reality" might be at least as valid if not more compelling than their own, the sad fact often is that their perspectival limitations prevent them from imagining what those other perspectives or outlooks might be.[27]

Mark Graber and his colleagues have observed that diagnostic errors become more likely when the level of uncertainty is high, the patient and his or her condition are unfamiliar, and the malady presents atypically, non-specifically, or with distracting comorbidities.[7,14] Also, we are generally biased toward making the "least costly error" over time.[28(p475)] After all, if the moral thrust of thinking about thinking is to reduce error, but not all errors can be prevented, then the ideal situation would be to develop safety practices and environments that allow only the "least costly error." But "costly" can have meanings that transcend patient suffering and the moral interests of metacognition.

I cannot resist remarking about "defensive medicine," such that in the interest of committing only the least costly errors, a physician may order numerous diagnostic tests, anticipating that none is likely to reveal anything significant but nevertheless wanting to leave no (costly) stone unturned. Yet, a 2016 study by Anupam Jena and his colleagues found that physicians who overutilize diagnostic tests are sued five times *less often* than physicians whose test ordering is more clinically reasonable or conservative.[29] So here, "costly" takes on liability connotations for the physician. Error theory would predict that when a large *fitness benefit,* or survival payoff, is associated with some performance or behavioral strategy, persons with decisional authority will favor that strategy, especially if they are in a position to benefit from the payoff.[28(p478)] Thus, while defensive medicine is known to be very costly to taxpayers, insured healthcare consumers, and health insurance companies, if doctors are convinced that it will diminish their liability, not to mention enhance their revenues, that perception of economic benefit will reinforce the practice. Furthermore, if physicians who practice defensive medicine are sued five times less often than those who don't, it would stand to reason that patients similarly value the overutilization of diagnostic tests. The physician who announces to a patient that he will leave no stone unturned in treating that patient's symptoms and so orders a bundle of likely low-yield tests may nevertheless endear himself to that patient, and, as Jena's study suggests, patients resist suing doctors they like. Paradoxically, then, defensive medicine turns out to be costly despite its avowed interest in making the least costly error.

Perhaps the greatest factor that compromises and explains why clinical reasoning can be so easily corrupted is the number of variables that affect it, given that clinical reasoning begins in a state of uncertainty. Indeed, a great problem in rendering care according to professional standards is when the patient's condition is complicated by numerous comorbidities that can obscure precisely which standards should be in play. As Richard Cook remarks in his interview, he rarely sees a patient with only one disease process. Moreover, thinking about thinking is difficult because not only are health professionals at the mercy of their own cognitive limitations and biases, but they have to contend with productivity pressures and economic incentives that affect their thinking in less than ideal ways. Thinking about thinking, then, must be supplemented by strategies and resources that not only detect and analyze knowledge shortcomings, but return that information to the clinician and his or her organization in ways that enable improvement. The following section explores recommendations and efforts that seek to use mindfulness to improve diagnostic and clinical reasoning.

Mindfulness

The literature on mindfulness typically characterizes it according to its two primary features: (1) a cultivated in-the-moment attentiveness to one's sensory experience and (2) a nonjudgmental attitude toward those thoughts and feelings that occur in consciousness and that can bias our perceptions.[8] One of the primary goals of mindfulness is to reduce the "noise" of intrusive sensory inputs that make our cognitive outputs less accurate in judgment and decision making and less enjoyable in living our lives.

Mindfulness (hereafter MF) is an important skill for realizing a foundational role in patient safety ethics. It is deeply related to a hypothesis that I explored in my earlier work on *medical narcissism*. I was intrigued by how a constellation of psychological factors that discourage humility—like fascination with perfect performance, poorly developed ego defenses in the presence of errors or mistakes, an exaggerated (sometimes sadomasochistically based) identification with one's work, an unreasonable and poorly calibrated sense of responsibility for a given outcome, and an indifference to the contributions and value of teamwork—compromise one's ethical behavior and the pursuit of logical, factually accurate, situationally sensitive approaches to decision making.[30] MF strategies address these psychological factors, among others, although like the pursuit of humility, these techniques can take a lifetime to master:

- Accepting that error commission is as an essential and inevitable part of learning and being human
- Developing a critical stance toward one's phenomenal and cognitive experience, such as the ability to appreciate perspective and the learning process, as well as awareness of memory and information synthesis limitations

- Developing a keen capacity to identify and regulate intrusive and un-productive thoughts and feelings
- Down-regulating ego-protective behaviors
- Practicing self-monitoring and self-auditing, that is, stepping outside oneself and watching oneself be oneself

For clinical scenarios, Croskerry has recommended

- learning the metacognitive strategies implicated in the previous bullet points;
- acquiring knowledge of errors that are common to specific interventions;
- identifying scenarios in which error is likely to occur, such as short staffing, incomplete documentation, easy to miss diagnoses, and so forth;
- applying "cognitive forcing strategies," that is, "[a] deliberate, conscious selection of a particular strategy in a specific situation to optimize decision making and avoid error"; and
- avoiding the temptation to minimize errors.[26(p115)]

Mindful practitioners believe that a more concentrated attention to the present moment's experience will relieve us of "self-interested" habits of mind—a common narcissistically based anxiety—that can derail the healthy pursuit of our professional and personal life goals. MF practice seeks to "purify" our immersion in the present and to encourage letting go of our self-esteem needs. An interesting collateral benefit is the deep and honest acceptance of being wrong.[31] Humility allows us to achieve a kind of self-neutrality, perhaps a kind of "self-forgetfulness," which allows us to absorb the content of the experience without the defensive responses that distort an accurate assessment of that experience's meaning.[30] Thus, the persistent practice of MF may result in better emotional regulation, less worry about future consequences, and a greater openness to feedback and coaching. A central objective in MF practice is that practitioners come to understand change, unpredictability, loss, suffering, failure, and other ego-deflating experiences of life as inevitable, instructive, and not as horrible or destructive as they might at first seem.

Dennis Novack's 1997 coauthored essay "Calibrating the Physician" offers the following question as encouraging a mindful approach to error commission.[32] What would it be like to respond to error with an attitude that is not encumbered with excessive defensiveness, anxiety, or arrogance so that I could consider the nature of my mistake; my beliefs about the mistake; the emotions I experienced in the aftermath of the mistake; how I coped with the mistake; and the changes I made in my practice as a result of the mistake? It seems that patient safety sensibilities would take a considerable leap forward if healthcare teams and their institutional leaders could answer these questions with what Michael and Abigail Lipson have called "a willed abandonment of self-interest."[33(p21)] In the following pages, I explore strategies based on or recalling MF for reducing diagnostic error and improving clinical reasoning and therefore the diagnostic process.

PART II: MINDFULNESS STRATEGIES FOR REDUCING DIAGNOSTIC ERROR AND FOR IMPROVING THE DIAGNOSTIC PROCESS

Before the IOM published its comprehensive report on diagnostic error in 2015, one of the better papers I came across on strategies for reducing rates of diagnostic error and improving clinical reasoning was published in 2010 by the Pennsylvania Patient Safety Authority (PPSA).[34] The PPSA is an 11-member state agency—whose personnel are appointed by the governor and state representatives—that receives incident reports of legislatively defined serious events and other adverse events. Although at the time the article appeared, the authority's taxonomy did not include a category for diagnostic error, the PPSA nevertheless reviewed 100 events related to error between June 2004 and November 2009. I've selected what I believe are the most salient findings and recommendations related to human factors and system improvements that bear on diagnostic errors.

1. Admit the reality of diagnostic and performance error. The report suggests that the language of "error" and "mistake" can be off-putting to health professionals, who might prefer a less accusatory vocabulary. Anecdotal evidence suggests that many clinicians are loath to use "error" language and instead prefer phrases like "There was a problem," "incident," or "therapeutic misadventure." The ethical problem arises, however, when these more benign-sounding terms obscure what really happened, that the cause of the harm was an error or an obvious departure from the standard of care. The PPSA report nevertheless goes on to point out that if the usual suspects in diagnostic error involve cognitive-processing issues, communication breakdowns, and system design problems, health professionals might feel less blamable and more willing to study "objective" factors, especially system-related ones, that can improve their diagnostic and reasoning processes.

Unfortunately, until feedback mechanisms are dramatically improved and healthcare institutions improve their work environments in ways that reduce diagnostic error traps and pitfalls, high rates of diagnostic error will likely continue. Indeed, it seems unrealistic for individuals to recognize and do something about their reasoning flaws when they have to use that very cognitive and emotional equipment to detect and grapple with them. Perhaps, then, an educational effort or program directed at mindfulness about diagnostic error would be better handled by the educational arms of residency programs or by medical malpractice carriers, whose interest in reducing diagnostic error is obvious. Indeed, among larger physician groups that self-insure and where a serious diagnostic error by one doctor might cause a considerable premium increase affecting all the physicians in the group, an interest in such education seems obvious.

The best time for such education to begin is early, especially in medical school and residency training, where clinical reasoning is in its formative stages. Remarkably, though, and attesting to the still nascent state of learning about diagnostic error, most medical schools and residency programs have no dedicated course on clinical reasoning. Later on in the careers of physicians, the literature suggests, they will only change their diagnostic approaches to *specific* symptom presentations rather than embark on a wholesale remodeling of their clinical reasoning behavior, as an MF approach might recommend.[11]

2. Learn metacognition and cognitive error traps. For staff expertise to develop, professionals need to pool their knowledge to identify where committing cognitive or diagnostic error is easy. In one of Croskerry's papers, he offers the following case scenario as illustrative of such pitfalls:

A 21-year-old man is brought to a trauma center by ambulance. He has been stabbed multiple times in the arms, chest, and head. He is in no significant distress. He is inebriated but cooperative. He has no dyspnea or shortness of breath; air entry is equal in both lungs; oxygen saturation, blood pressure, and pulse are all within normal limits. The chest laceration over his left scapula is deep but on exploration does not appear to penetrate the chest cavity. Nevertheless, there is concern that the chest cavity and major vessels may have been penetrated. Ultrasonography shows no free fluid in the chest; a chest film appears normal, with no pneumothorax; and an abdominal series is normal, with no free air. There is considerable discussion between the resident and the attending physician regarding the management of posterior chest stab wounds, but eventually agreement is reached that computed tomography (CT) of the chest is not indicated. The remaining lacerations are cleaned and sutured, and the patient is discharged home in the company of his friend. Five days later, he presents to a different hospital reporting vomiting, blurred vision, and difficulty concentrating. A CT of his head reveals the track of a knife wound penetrating the skull and several inches into the brain.[35(p2446)]

Croskerry suggests that "anchoring" and "search satisficing" were the cognitive biasing culprits here, as the resident and attending staff focused on the chest wound and failed to conduct a sufficient search to rule out other significant injuries. Cognitive scientists have identified more than 100 of these pitfalls that affect our reasoning and judgments, so it is a wonder we are not wrong more often. But therein lies a trap: Because health professionals' clinical judgments, perceptions, and decisions are usually right or at least justifiable, they can easily lose the capacity to maintain a critical attitude toward them. Not only is doing so effortful, but when one is rushed by production quotas and time pressures, the quality of a clinically sound workup can be degraded, so that misses, incorrect attributions, false assumptions, and faulty logic become virtually inevitable. Here, little attention is paid to whether an error might be "least costly" or very costly; rather, there is only the reality of production pressures.

Croskerry and others recommend implementing *cognitive forcing* strategies, which are essentially techniques of vigilance and "de-biasing."[26] To acquire such a practice and mental orientation, the practitioner must admit the fallibility of his or her judgment; know where the error traps lie for a specific diagnostic challenge; detect whether environmental variables are in play (such as fatigue, inexperienced staff, too many patients to be seen, and especially feelings of uncertainty over the patient's symptom presentation); and then review and implement good clinical reasoning per the situation at hand. One of the most prominent problems is that the more seasoned the practitioner, the more likely he or she will rely on first impressions and be so convinced of their accuracy that the diagnostic search is terminated: "[B]ecause reliance on nonanalytical reasoning tends to increase with experience, it is possible that physicians with many years of clinical practice may be even more susceptible to availability bias than second-year residents

. . . [T]he tendency to diagnose cases through pattern recognition increases with clinical experience."[12(p1202)]

These comments recall James Reason's observation that patient safety is a guerilla war that the professional will eventually lose, because the kind of hypervigilance that characterizes a cognitive-forcing stance seems impossible to consistently maintain.[18] This is why reducing diagnostic and clinical reasoning errors is, somewhat paradoxically, a collective effort that entails multiple reasoners and observers, environments that utilize good reasoning, user-friendly technological support, and an administrative dedication and energy to making system changes informed by mistakes. The challenge is relentless and endless.

3. Extend the clinician's mindfulness with technological support for clinical reasoning. Neurophilosophers have proposed and studied an intriguing idea called the "extended mind thesis."[36] Although these scholars are interested in the more esoteric dimensions of this notion, such as the composition of mental states and what kind of content mental states need to qualify as mental states, people actually started "extending" their minds when they began tying a string around their finger to remind them to do something. The value of devices that extend (often by substituting for) our powers of perception (e.g., using video surveillance), attention (e.g., with automatic pilot), and information retrieval and synthesis (e.g., with computers) seems inarguable. But these devices are also mindfulness assets, which the PPSA advocates, for example, a greater use of clinical decision support systems such as web-based applications, computer-assisted feature mapping, data visualization tools, diagnostic checklists, and technology that supplies readily available clinical guidelines and clinical algorithms.

Perhaps the most familiar technological innovation that could significantly reduce the frequency of diagnostic error is the electronic medical record (EMR). For example, in the sulfa drug allergy case discussed in chapter 1 (Case 1.1), had the EMR been programmed to transfer the nurse's or the pulmonologist's notation of the patient's drug allergy directly to the drug allergy drop-down box, the patient's death might have been averted. Indeed, the EMR of the future will likely direct the health professional's attention or diagnostic curiosity to this or that symptom cluster, finding, or pattern; recommend an additional diagnostic test or a need for a consult; alert the clinician to contraindications (which some already do); or remind the clinician that individuals with the patient's symptoms are also at high risk for X or Y or Z, which might need to be examined or might automatically require a consultation.[21] (See the interview with Bob Wachter in chapter 9.)

Unfortunately, EMRs have been beset by design and implementation problems that continue to witness a tremendous volume of complaints from clinicians.[9(pp5.10-5.13)] But consider a remarkable 1998 study of Dutch physicians, in which physician participants were able to enter their diagnostic findings and impressions directly into a computer, push a button, and learn what the computer's diagnostic program was differentially or probabilistically "thinking" at any point during the information-gathering and synthesizing process.[37] What surprised the investigators was that despite the physicians' eagerness to learn what the program was "thinking" (that is, they pushed the button often), the computer's "judgment" *almost never caused them to revise their own clinical impressions.* Even as the physicians were in the process of formulating an opinion, not to mention once their minds were made up, the computer-generated diagnoses—differential diagnoses that the computer could offer at any point in the data-entry process— virtually never altered the physicians' diagnostic opinions or their level of confidence. The researchers concluded that the physicians' keen interest in learning what the computer was registering was motivated not as a reasoning check but as a reasoning *confirmation.* In other words, a physician's eagerness "to reveal the system's list of diagnoses has little to do with a critical attitude towards his own judgement, but has everything to do with his anxiety to have his diagnostic ideas confirmed."[37(p98)] If this finding is generalizable, how long will that professional stubbornness.persist? We now have every reason to expect a steady stream of artificially intelligent medical and diagnostic devices and supporting technologies to arise over the coming decades. If current information technologies can beat the best human contestants on television game shows and play chess better than any of the world's grandmasters, it seems only a matter of time until various AI technologies will replace many human operators, especially in activities like interpreting and processing information related to radiologic images or laboratory specimens.[38(pp12-13)]

Tejal Gandhi and her colleagues directed some excellent commonsense attention to the need for "tickler" and test-result-tracking systems to keep patients and physicians on a reliable schedule. Of 181 medical malpractice claims that Gandhi's group studied involving a missed or delayed diagnoses in an ambulatory setting, the mean interval between when the diagnosis should have been made and when it was actually made was 465 days, with a median of 303 days (and a range of 36 to 681 days).[25] Had communication technologies been available to contact the patient directly or through a physician's office for clinical updates, some of these delays might not have occurred. It seems highly likely that technologies of the near future will be doing something of that sort. Such systems could provide professionals with checklists or prompts on where to look, what to ask, what to test, what information to gather or tests to order, which findings are likely to prove highly significant and which ones less so, and what should be the features of an adequate follow-up plan.[39]

In 2013, Robert El-Kareh, Omar Hasan, and Gordon Schiff presented an excellent overview of the current state of diagnostic health information technologies (HITs) currently on the market.[40] They noted that HITs fell into the following categories:

- HITs that aid in information gathering, such as automated patient interviewing that assists in or complements a physician's or nurse's history taking
- Technologies that graphically represent numerical data, leading to reduced review times and greater ease in representing data that answer clinical questions as well as helping ensure that items don't get overlooked
- Tools that provide diagnostic checklists and remind the clinician of "don't miss" diagnoses
- Screen displays that provide probability rankings (or diagnostic weightings) of differential diagnoses or that use "clinical prediction rules" that rank "the likelihood of diagnoses based on sets of clinical systems, signs or test results"[40(p5)]
- Electronic products such as "infobuttons" that provide context-specific links from clinical impressions or to reference systems in recognized databases, the latter tool directly linking with the patient's EMR so that the physician doesn't have to exit it and search another database
- Tools that alert clinicians to patients' need for screening tests, early disease detection, or follow-up visits
- Telemedicine devices that facilitate diagnostic collaborations and expert consultations
- Technologies that facilitate feedback and insight into diagnostic performance

What is unsettling about the authors' ultimate findings, however, is this observation: "Overall, we found that progress in diagnostic HIT has been slow and incremental with few significant 'game-changing' approaches emerging in the last decade."[40(p7)] But perhaps this isn't as surprising at it seems considering that to implement such technologies, healthcare leadership must be convinced that the technology not only enables "significantly improved" outcomes (whose measurements can be controversial) but is also affordable. In addition, it must be reasonably user friendly in terms of integration within clinical workflow, operational manipulation, user comprehension, and ease of maintenance and updating. Making such determinations and then committing to them takes enormous time and effort, which may be in short organizational supply; thus, one of the authors concluded, "[T]he field of diagnostic health information technology is still in its early stages and there has been minimal development over the past decade in various promising realms . . . [F]ew tools and systems have been shown to improve diagnosis in actual clinical settings."[40(p8)]

And then we have Richard Cook's rueful comment that with innovation comes new forms of failure.[41] An AI diagnostic technology that recommends a patient be worked up for a half-dozen presumptive ailments may be rejected as economically counterproductive if the tests aren't covered by the patient's insurer, but the physician's failure to accommodate that technology's treatment recommendation might, at some point in the future of AI, result in a malpractice action. If these AI technologies become widely adopted, the threat of medical malpractice litigation virtually demands that new standards of practice be developed defining the nature of what a "reasonable judgment" will resemble in an age when not only are physicians and AI systems working side by side, but physicians occasionally cede decisional authority to the system.[42]

4. *Improve internal data-gathering systems on errors in clinical reasoning.* An adjunct to improving technological support for system operators' decision making is to improve how we understand MF lapses. Consider how easily diagnostic errors evade detection and never become a source for learning. The professional may have no idea he or she is missing something; many months might go by before the diagnostic oversight or error is discovered; a correction might be made by a different physician, with an error report that never reaches the index physician; the patient's symptoms might resolve on their own; or the patient might move away or die.[18] Also, whether a diagnostic error in fact occurred or a physician missed something that any physician would ordinarily notice might be debatable. These possibilities imply the need for formal, perhaps institutionally mediated, diagnostic expertise featuring multiple personnel who can improve patient safety by

studying, adjudicating, and disseminating information on diagnostic mishaps and then fostering system changes. For that to happen, though, rich databases on diagnostic error must be developed. Also, leadership should make diagnostic error and clinical reasoning top priorities in professional education and quality assurance planning, in addition to risk managers modifying their internal reporting systems to track and analyze diagnostic errors and their events.

5. Improve feedback to clinicians. Mindfulness cannot advance without training, and one of the most obvious and perhaps most effective training techniques in healthcare is feedback. In Jack Ende's classic 1983 essay, "Feedback in Clinical Medical Education," he quotes Norbert Weiner's definition of feedback as "the control of a system by reinserting into the system the results of its performance."[43(p777)] This literature represents feedback as not so much judgment or evaluation than formative information that "highlights the dissonance between the intended result and the actual result, thereby providing impetus for change."[43(p777)] In contrast to judgment, good feedback sharply focuses on the technical details of performance or on how someone performs this or that task rather than on his or her attitude, commitment, values, professional growth, and so forth.[43]

One would think persons executing tasks with the potential to seriously harm others would welcome feedback—indeed, would aggressively seek it out. Ende reported, though, that many residents in his day were resistant to feedback, as they "seemed to employ a whole barrage of defenses for dealing with criticism from superiors . . . [Y]oung professionals develop the tendency to fix their standards of performance in such a way as to resist efforts by others to change them."[43(p779)] Possibly, though, the "feedback" these residents received was poorly delivered, because the literature is keen to note that good feedback ought disturb only the most emotionally sensitive of trainees.[44] Good feedback is not evaluative in the sense of telling individuals how well they performed (e.g., "That was pretty good") but focuses more on correcting or improving performance proficiency (e.g., "You wanted to order medicine X for this patient, but X is contraindicated because of Z"). It's possible that the residents of Ende's generation developed psychological defenses because they received feedback in ways that embarrassed and humiliated them. If so, that is lamentable, because performance research, as well as common sense, indicates that improvement reaches a point where further progress is all but impossible without good feedback.[45(pS34)]

A major impediment to giving constructive feedback is the teacher's not wanting to hurt the listener's feelings, so that he or she avoids sounding critical and responds only with positives or encouragement, while some instructors give no feedback at all. Perhaps these instructors are anxious about receiving a defensive reply that will upset them. Furthermore, much of clinical teaching is performed by people who are not trained educators.[46] But as long as the feedback is specific to performance or technique and is delivered in a way that improves the listener's skill set, as a good sports coach does, the listener should be grateful for the information. After all, learners oftentimes can't identify their weaknesses, much less improve them, such that without accurate and timely feedback, the likelihood of that improvement vectors to zero.

Unfortunately, the absence of good feedback among healthcare professionals is pervasive and systemic. In 2008, Gordon Schiff wrote on how this absence typically affects diagnostic errors:

> [C]linicians learn about their diagnostic successes or failures in various ad hoc ways (e.g., a knock on the door from a server with a malpractice subpoena; a medical resident learning, upon bumping into a surgical resident in the hospital hallway[,] that a patient he/she cared for has been readmitted; a radiologist accidentally stumbling upon an earlier chest x-ray of a patient with lung cancer and noticing a nodule that had been overlooked). Physicians lack systematic methods for calibrating diagnostic decisions based on feedback from their outcomes. Worse yet, organizations have no way to learn about the thousands of collective diagnostic decisions that are made each day—information that could allow them to both improve overall performance as well as better hear the voices of the patients living with their outcomes.[44(pS38)]

Without feedback on one's errors, "no news is good news." Because Dr. Smith hears next to nothing about her reasoning and diagnostic acumen, she will assume them adequate if not superlative. Considering how the absence of negative feedback reinforces the comfortable feelings attached to a clinician's personal conviction of adequacy, the paucity of good feedback becomes all the more alarming: "[W]eak or ambiguous feedback contributes to the situation by preventing physicians from learning when their self-confirming routines are inappropriate, inaccurate, or dangerous."[44(pS36)]

For good reading on improving feedback, readers can study the papers referenced above as well as those by Gigante, Dell, and Sharkey; Cantillon and Sargeant; and, especially, Brinko and Ramani and Krackov.[47-50] A general suggestion among these works is that giving feedback should be based on the teacher's direct observation of the learner's performance and that feedback sessions should be formally scheduled so that they do not take the learner by surprise. More than one paper recommends delivering feedback as you would build layers of a sandwich: Begin with a positive comment, then elaborate on an area of improvement (more than one paper recommends discussing only one performance parameter at a time), and end with a positive comment. Seek the learner's self-assessment and always create a detailed plan for improvement. Ramani and Krackov note, "Feedback initiated solely or jointly by learners was seen as more instructive than that initiated mainly by teachers"; thus, the ideal goal is engaged communication that culminates with the learner's gaining greater confidence in his or her technical skill building or recognizing where room for improvement exists and learning what constitutes that improvement.[50(p789)]

Mindfulness: A Summation

I keep returning to Herbert Simon's account of "bounded rationality" and how it speaks to the nature of absent knowledge in the professional-patient encounter. Neither the professional nor the patient has anything approaching comprehensive knowledge of all that is pertinent or relevant to what is going on—the etiology of the patient's symptoms (and whether the professional should know that etiology or not), the psychological factors that affect their therapeutic relationship, the cognitive traps and pitfalls that confront each of them, whether diagnostic standards are in place that should be strictly (or loosely) followed, and how their values and understandings of what is "reasonable" to do will affect moving forward. The ubiquity of knowledge gaps and lacunae is nicely evoked by Schiff's wondering what having a "partial response" to treatment ultimately means.[44] Does it mean that the treatment was only "partially" correct in assisting the patient's improvement and that another, better treatment was available? Or does it mean that the treatment was entirely inefficacious, with the patient's partial improvement owing to something else? Or that a "part" of the patient's illness responded and another part didn't? While it's entirely possible that no treatment would have effected a satisfying outcome, how would we know this without adequate evidence, which may or may not be available?

What we do know is that many studies corroborate a high rate of diagnostic errors—roughly 10 to 30 percent in general—including autopsy studies noting the prevalence of diagnostic errors by way of misses or major autopsy findings that had not been addressed by the patients' treatments. For example, in 2003 Kaveh Shojania and his colleagues reviewed more than 50 autopsy studies and speculated that in an average hospital, 8 to 24 percent of cases were being treated with an incorrect diagnosis or with one that entirely missed the patient's primary problem.[51] Granted, the legitimacy of error findings from autopsy studies are questionable because they provide the error rate only in patients who die. Also, as Western health professionals perform fewer autopsies, the ones that are performed are likely to be on the more challenging cases, where there might be a higher probability of error (or where error was easier to commit), thus raising concerns over their representativeness. Nevertheless, these autopsy studies are sobering as they continue to suggest high rates of errors over the decades, at least among the patient cohort likely to be autopsied.

What we are ethically left with are three areas of interest in the mindfulness of clinical reasoning and knowledge processing: (1) the majority of cases, in which health professionals are justifiably on the right track in treating patients' maladies based on a "sufficient" or "reasonable" degree of evidence to warrant their plan and the absence of system malfunctions; (2) a brace of difficult cases in which the correct diagnosis eludes physicians' epistemic grasp, and their judgment is hit or miss; and (3) the rather significant number of studies, such as the ones reported above, that suggest the occurrence of too many error-caused adverse events resulting from cognitive imperfections mixing with system flaws. As the first two kinds of decision making are ethically unproblematic, assuming the clinician and his or her support system are doing all they reasonably can, our ethical attention should focus on the third group, in which the patient harms are precipitated by error and thus, in principle, preventable.

At the current moment, the US healthcare system frequently delivers astonishing successes, such as the evolution of cancer and musculoskeletal therapies, not to mention basic public health improvements that, over the last 60 years, have prevented uncountable numbers of deaths worldwide. But we have also evolved a delivery system that continues to suffer from a remarkable inertia in learning from its mistakes and making system improvements. This inertia suggests that deeper underlying factors are militating against safety—underscoring the popular adage that systems deliver precisely what they are designed to deliver, but also implying that relevant system change is likely difficult and costly. Furthermore, persistently high harm-causing error rates might stem from the deterioration of many healthcare organizations into "cultures of low expectations," where the pressure and demands for revenue generation have forced personnel to cut corners and take shortcuts whenever possible, and where the acquisition of medical and organizational knowledge, along with the will to act on their patient safety lessons, remains stunted.[52(p829)] In addition, the furious pace of technologically driven changes in healthcare environments may exceed the psychomotor ability of personnel to implement them.[37]

Accordingly, this chapter's exploration of mindfulness illustrates the following points:

- Admitting the reality of error requires that professionals have the courage to accept the unpleasantness of their fallibility and aggressively seek to improve their patient safety skill set. If they were thoroughly patient centered, they'd want to preserve only the correct and ethical parts of their performance. The rest they would want to replace with better. Thus, they'd ultimately need something on the order of expert teachers or coaches who could point out skill deficits and explain ways to improve.[53] How do we effect the attitudinal change that's required for this? Two good strategies are to use available technologies to reveal errors and to improve feedback.

- Health professionals will continue to have a difficult time admitting errors. As I note in chapter 7, they hesitate to complete incident reports and often do not view diagnostic error as something to report the way they would a wrong-side surgery or medication error. Diagnostic errors may seem like uniquely personal or "soft" errors. They may appear less onerous or alarming than a wrong-side surgery or a medication error, even though risk managers would want to know about them all.

- The mindful practitioner needs a knowledge base on error traps and system flaws, and health facilities need to commit to teaching these topics. We clearly need a national effort to collect and promulgate information on uniquely challenging types of diagnoses.

- Mindfulness needs to be taught as a skill set. It requires knowledge of one's cognitive vulnerabilities, attentional and focusing techniques, empathy, redirecting feelings from unhelpful or disorienting feelings to constructive and positive ones, and engaging patients and families in the diagnostic process. In line with this, the diagnostic process should occasionally allow a *collective* intelligence, whereby the diagnostician stops feeling his or her individuality so intensely and invites multiple others to join in the diagnostic effort.

- If these recommendations sound too difficult, we might look to technology to improve clinical reasoning. Current technologies emphasize thoroughness and differential diagnoses. Perhaps the electronic record of the not-too-distant future will alert physicians to the possibility of improbable diagnoses, remind them of former patients whose diagnoses they missed, or discern important trends or patterns in the patient's medical history that are clinically meaningful. How these technological possibilities will be received as they become available is anyone's guess. But if they are spectacularly successful and considerably surpass human standards, insurance companies might strongly encourage their use with premium-reduction incentives.

These thoughts return us to the extended mind, or perhaps *extended mindfulness*, thesis. Patient safety policies are as much a product of our technologies, cultural attitudes, and values as they are a product of scientifically produced knowledge. Because the latter seems considerably driven by the former, an ethically essential task of mindfulness is for health professionals to look deeply into themselves, examine their own needs and worries, consider how their work environments shape expectations, and determine what should be retained as well as given up in the interests of patient safety. Let us hope that whatever clinical practices and system operations materialize, they will be ethically defensible and make healthcare delivery safer.

Interview with Pat Croskerry

Pat Croskerry, MD, PhD, is a professor in the Dalhousie University Division of Medical Education in Halifax and director of the Critical Thinking Program. He has published more than 80 journal articles and 30 book chapters on patient safety and clinical decision making, in addition to giving more than 500 presentations locally, nationally, and internationally. His research has focused on clinical decision making, with emphasis on the diagnostic process. Croskerry established the first Canadian Symposium on Patient Safety and has served on various organizing committees for conferences addressing the problem of diagnostic error. He was a recent member of the US IOM's Committee on Diagnostic Error in Health Care and served as a board member of the Canadian Patient Safety Institute. Croskerry has received numerous awards for his work in patient safety, among them the Royal College of Physicians and Surgeons of Canada Speaker Award (2006), the John Ruedy Award for Innovation in

Box 3.1. Characteristics of Mindful Practice

- Uses cognitive-forcing strategies, that is, strategies that seek to offset human fallibility by making error commission harder, especially by taking the time to deliberate and reflect more thoroughly, such as by asking, "What do I not want to miss? What am I assuming? Am I fair to all the evidence? Do I need a consult? Am I using a checklist? What are likely alternative diagnoses and treatments?"
- Is self-critical, objectifying oneself in order to observe and evaluate performance in the work environment, while wondering, "How do I appear to those outside me?"
- Actively seeks feedback on performance
- Teaches principles of clinical reasoning
- Practices being patient and thorough as well as using decision support technologies
- Is extremely sensitive to and self-aware about cognitive traps, such as memory limitations, information-processing weaknesses, biases, and so on
- Encourages and participates in team learning, reflection, self-criticism, and knowledge acquisition
- Maintains awareness of what's happening in the performance environment
- Practices critical curiosity and openness, especially in moments that seem atypical, odd, or unexpected
- Resists unreasonable optimism
- Often returns to basics and appreciates the need to begin over—that is, practices the "beginner's mind"
- Is humble in the face of personal flaws, weaknesses, and inadequacies
- Demonstrates compassion and openness toward oneself and others
- Is willing to be in the moment
- Commits to lifelong learning, including coaching, practicing via simulation devices, and teaching others
- Reviews, studies, and remembers botched cases[6,54,55]

Medical Education (2006), and the James S. Todd Memorial Award for Patient Safety Research (2002).

JB: Pat, thanks so much for doing this interview with me. You are one of the foremost scholars in the area of diagnostic error and clinical reasoning; you've authored dozens of papers appearing in the highest impact medical journals on these topics; and you're constantly traveling the world speaking to medical and clinical groups on how we might reduce diagnostic error and improve clinical reasoning. So my first question is, Are you seeing a positive change over the last ten years towards lessening the rates of diagnostic errors, or is the challenge of improving diagnostic reasoning still too daunting for most teaching institutions and healthcare delivery systems to take on?

PC: Well, when I started getting interested in this area around 1999, the medical community was quite naïve about the subject, which is amazing because when you think about it, clinical reasoning is the most important thing we do. So, what should have happened is for the medical community to say, "Well, given the importance of clinical reasoning, we have to make sure we understand it and teach it appropriately." But when I was in training, I wasn't taught it, nor were my colleagues. Historically, medical teachers simply assumed that students would pick up clinical reasoning skills osmotically, I suppose, by just being around faculty and watching and absorbing how they do it. But now we are taking a much more informed and, frankly, scientific, or empirical, approach to clinical reasoning, which there is no question will continue. For example, I was in Great Britain just a few weeks ago and learned that a consortium of medical schools have banded together and acronymized their group as CReME—standing for "clinical reasoning in medical education" (they had to use an *e* for the middle letter instead of an *i* for the obvious reason). Of course, there is the Society for the Improvement of Diagnosis in Medicine as well. And there are more publications and studies appearing in our clinical journals than one can read. So, I would answer your question from the vantage point of 2016 with a resounding "yes"; we have begun to make real progress.

JB: It seems to me that there must be a real attitudinal change involving humility for this to happen, because it forces physicians to face the limits and imperfections of their cognition.

PC: That reminds me of one of the first papers I wrote, entitled "The Cognitive Imperative," which I submitted in 2000 to a top journal—so that was about six years before Jerry Groopman's book on *How Doctors Think* came out. The paper was summarily rejected, with the reviewer comments being, as I recall, almost patronizing, as in "How dare you suggest that doctors can't think?" They were almost insulted that I would suggest that there might be flaws in physicians' thinking.

JB: And, of course, we can look back on the history of the reluctance of physicians to admit and discuss their medical errors as a contributing factor.

PC: Errors were so little discussed 20 years ago that you could get the impression that clinicians didn't make any. But, as you know, I came into medicine with a background in experimental psychology, and I was astounded to see physicians doing things to patients that I was trained not to do with laboratory rats; I mean not following protocols or standards or rules very closely or sometimes not at all. When I asked residents or attending physicians about it, they would just shrug and say, "That's the way we do it here." Now, I'm not saying that physicians are insensitive people, but those days were rather different from today because back then, patients wanted their doctors to look and sound confident and in control. A physician who said, "Well, it could be this, it could be that"—which today would be something we'd recommend in nonobvious situations—would probably bother many patients back then who want[ed] to think of their doctors as infallible. You might say that doctors back then were being manipulated by their patients' need for certainty, and so they delivered by frequently effecting an overconfident manner, which their patients seemed to like. Also, that attitude and behavior may have strengthened a placebo effect of the clinician-patient relationship.

JB: I recall that when I started studying medical ethics about 35 years ago, physicians would commonly say that you can't say "I don't know" to a patient's question. Clearly, both sides were insecure about human fallibility. I sense that today, things have changed considerably, so that, from what I read, patients and family members appreciate the clinician's expression of not knowing or of uncertainty as a sign of his or her trustworthiness. I want to think they have developed the maturity and understanding to realize that their clinicians are not omniscient.

PC: However, there is something to the phenomenon of patients wanting "the simple truth" of their maladies. They might not want a detailed or in-depth account of what is going on—which the physician might not be able to truthfully supply—but many will want a kind of bottom line, so to speak, as in "How serious is this?" Or "How worried should I be about this?" There is a sense in which many patients don't want to think too hard, and they want their doctor to give them the basic picture of what is clinically going on.

JB: And to me, this says something interesting about the transformation of knowledge of medicine, at least as it is transmitted from the professional to the knowledge consumer: that we've given up a somewhat adolescent fantasy of thinking our physicians know everything for something more reasonable, but we still expect to get something approximating the truth from the medical community.

PC: Which, of course, is not unreasonable to ask.

JB: No, it isn't. Pat, I want to go back to your initial interest with reasoning errors in medicine and talk about the role of feedback, or the lack of it, that continues to pervade medicine. Someone said that if physicians got feedback on their missed or errant diagnoses the way weather people get feedback on their mistakes, we'd all be more appreciative about the need to study clinical reasoning.

PC: I think the problem is a virtually universal one. For example, we have to do evaluations at the end of students' rotations, and sometimes you just check the boxes on the form, but the people who run the program say, "Look, the students want feedback and an informed evaluation." In fact, if the human brain is an exquisite machine that nevertheless requires occasional calibration, then if you don't tell the machine how it's doing, don't expect any improvement. It's like putting a thermostat in a room and setting it to keep the room temperature at 70 degrees but not equipping the thermostat with a way to tell how hot or cold the room is. That would be ridiculous. So without feedback to human beings, the whole principle of calibrating behavior to adapt to the environment would be undermined. But people don't like giving feedback. If done properly, however, such that it's not judgmental but purely informative, it will further the calibration of the learner's judgment. It's exactly the right thing to do. Yet, I'm afraid lots of supervisors don't give good feedback because they are afraid of offending their students. So, they don't do a good job largely because they don't have the skills.

JB: I recall reading some papers where residents lamented not getting good feedback, which is the one thing they really wanted.

PC: Yes, but I've known institutions to start a feedback program where clinicians are taught good feedback techniques. But like so many well-intentioned programs, after a few months it kind of drops off and people forget about it. This is really a job for leadership to sustain a program like that, because left to their own devices, many of the faculty will stop doing it.

JB: So let's switch gears because I want to ask you about something that has fascinated me for a long time: the switch that goes on in a physician's clinical reasoning approach from medical school to, say, midcareer. From what I've learned, as that journey proceeds, the physician's diagnostic reasoning changes from a Bayesian analytic reasoning to a prototypical kind of symptom recognition and treatment approach. And, for the most part, that's fine, because physicians usually get it right. But not always, which is the problem. So, how do you get a physician who's been out in the field for 20 or 30 years to go back to those days of analytical reasoning and forswear the quick and easy and largely effortless kind of diagnostic approach typical of prototype thinking?

PC: I think what you have to do is to raise awareness of the actual processes going on. So we teach the dual-processing System 1 and 2 models in medical training. And when you're a medical student, you're virtually entirely in System 2, and you will gradually over the years move into System 1 and use it probably 95 percent of the time. The problem is, though, that experts remain vulnerable; 95 percent of the time, however, you will do absolutely fine, but sometimes you will fall into a trap and be, frankly, humiliated. So experts need to know their vulnerabilities, and novices have to know theirs, but those recognitions are quite different. Novices have to learn enough to get them from System 2 to System 1, but once they are there, they have to learn that this is not entirely safe ground. It's very much like learning to drive a car such that after a while, you no longer have to think about how much distance you need to keep between yourself and other drivers, how fast you can go, and all those things. But in medicine, you have to realize that a 95 percent success rate using System 1 cognition simply isn't good enough. In our emergency room department, we see 100 patients a day, so you can see how in a very short period of time, that 5 percent of patients who have suffered missed or delayed or mistaken diagnoses will add up. So experts need to be mindful of what they are doing. What mindfulness does is help us be more careful among that 5 percent where you might get it very wrong. In fact, classical training from the Eastern traditions in mindfulness is often helpful in detecting the biases or heuristical pitfalls in System 1 reasoning, which also goes under the name "cognitive debiasing."

JB: Do you think there's a moment in medical training when we can introduce students to this?

PC: At Dalhousie, we introduce students to the nature of reasoning very early, and many of them ask, "What does this have to do with my becoming a doctor?" to which we say, "It has everything to do with it." But you have to be patient because they're concentrating on anatomy and physiology and all those things. By the time they're finishing their training, though, they understand how important it is to know these things. So we teach it right from the very beginning.

JB: So, what are the prospects for the kind of mindfulness that you're advocating for today's clinical workplace, where health professionals are under such production pressures and where, I think, their baseline cognitive self-perception, their feeling of themselves, is one of mild but persisting anxiety?

PC: So that is a question which I get asked frequently. I think part of the problem is that doctors have dug their own grave. People say to me, "Well, it's all very fine this mindfulness stuff that you talk about, but how can we complete all our work given the enormous constraints we're under? We don't have time to step back and analyze our thinking." And I say to them that doctors have to stop agreeing to stay on the treadmill. But administration wants doctors to run on that treadmill at a rate that is unsafe. If you told a bank teller who is working with another customer to just sign this form because you can't wait—which happens all the time in medicine—he'd tell you to get back in line. Now, we know that those production pressures lead to error. So you have to say to management that we no longer want to work in these conditions because doing so means we will have to work in a System 1 mode, which is dangerous. In my opinion, doctors should challenge the work environment that administrators have created.

The second thing doctors can do is disabuse themselves of the idea that saying to themselves, "Hmm, what else can this be? Have I missed something glaring? Is there something else I need to check before I sign off on this?" takes all that long. It's a very critical juncture when you are preparing to sign off, because when you do, thinking stops. And I've found that if you pause and ask yourself these questions, which might require an extra 20 seconds in your thinking, it can be enough to alert you to an assumption that may be unjustified. So, I don't think that's a significant hardship. What can and should happen is that the physician should automatically add that pause-and-reflect recalibration to his or her thinking. And once you get into the habit of doing that, you can do it quickly and effectively without halting the process.

JB: So, Pat, let me end with this question: What are you most excited about in the field of clinical reasoning? I'm especially wondering what your take is on the new diagnostic technologies that are out there or teaching prospects for our medical students and residents. Where do you think the field is going in the next 5 or 10 years and what are you most excited about?

PC: I think there are two big things coming. One is the IBM Watson, which will handle big data, natural language interaction with the machine, and so on. Of course, one problem is that no machine is better than the information going into it. Also, and somewhat unfortunately, a machine has to be a super machine to compensate for human error. So if a patient is talking to a computer and not giving an accurate account, then we're going to be no better for it. Also, we have to be very careful as to how we're going to control that kind of technology and not allow it to substitute for things that humans do better, like taking a good history and physical. So, one of my major concerns is about the quality of the interface between the patient and the machine.

The second thing is that Dalhousie is the first medical school, I think, to have a course solely dedicated to critical thinking. And I think that's a major step forward—that is, our acknowledging that physician thinking is worth having a special university program dedicated to it. We have a critical thinking website; we teach students about logical fallacies; and we also teach them about the kinds of cognitive pitfalls that await physicians. We have some faculty describe cases that have gone wrong—and these physicians are highly experienced—and we show students how a doctor can make a mess of something. So, we want to get the students to the point where they can analyze the case and identify the cognitive errors that led to things going wrong and how they could have been avoided.

JB: Actually, that's the thrust of this book. I want to use errors and mistakes that have occurred in medical malpractice as learning examples of how things can go wrong. Sort of "look at what this case can teach us or suggest to us about improving patient safety and clinical thinking."

PC: We have something called the "Cognitive Autopsy Manual," which is a manual for students that describes 30 cases, all of which went bad. So we provide the student with an "autopsy" of the cognition that accounted for the error. We're probably going to publish that soon. And I and a group of my colleagues are going to be bringing about a new book soon on diagnostic reasoning that, frankly, ten years ago, and prior to Jerry Groopman's book, would have been unimaginable. So, it's tremendously exciting to be doing this work now.

JB: Oh, there's one last thing I want to ask you: electronic health records. I know many physicians positively hate them, but I also know that there's some literature where physicians are sounding cautiously optimistic that electronic health records may improve patient safety quite a bit. What's your impression?

PC: Well, you'll find a lot of people critical of the electronic health record, but I do agree that it has a huge potential for providing benefits for decision making, like giving accurate feedback in a timely fashion, recognizing data trends, immediate access to previous test, et cetera. But you have to have people designing those things who recognize the interface needs of humans and machines. They have to make it easy and reliable to use, and they mustn't allow shortcuts and gaming to occur. I think in the long run, it can have enormous benefits, but getting there will require time and patience.

JB: Wonderful. Pat, thanks so much for this.

PC: My pleasure.

4   Compliance

> When new technologies are used to eliminate well-understood system
> failures or to gain high precision performance, they often introduce new
> pathways to large scale, catastrophic failures. Not uncommonly, these
> new, rare catastrophes have even greater impact than those eliminated by
> the new technology.
>
> Richard Cook[1(p3)]

Chapter Overview: The chapter begins with a characterization of
deviance as an intentional "practice variation" in the form of a departure
from an established rule, regulation, or standard—in other words, deviance
when the system operator's compliance is required. I then offer examples
of deviating practices and discuss the fact that such deviations will occur for
long periods before one of them is implicated in a disaster. I then explore
why such deviations occur and why they persist. The chapter concludes
with a list of remediation strategies (see box 4.1).

COMPLIANCE FAILURES AND NORMALIZING DEVIANCE

Over the last decade, hospital safety personnel have gradually become dis-
abused of a long-standing but incorrect belief—that harm-causing medical
errors, like wrong-side surgeries or retained surgical instruments, result
from a single individual doing something inexplicably stupid. Instead, contemporary research on megadisasters like Chernobyl, the space shuttles
Challenger and *Columbia*, Bhopal, and any number of patient care catastrophes has consistently shown that accidents like them require (1) multiple
people (2) committing multiple, often seemingly innocuous, mistakes that
(3) breach an organization's fail-safe mechanisms, defenses, or safety nets
resulting in (4) serious harm or disaster.[1-6] In other words, mistakes like failing to check or record a lab finding, ordering the wrong drug, or entering
a lab finding in the wrong patient's chart are usually not enough to guarantee an occurrence of harm. The recipe for disaster additionally requires
these errors, lapses, or mistakes *to go unattended, unappreciated, or unresolved*

for an extended period. Harm-causing errors therefore result from *active errors* intermingling with *latent errors*, like flaws or weaknesses in a system's defenses that allow the former to breach those defenses, reach patients, and cause harm.[5]

Remarkably, the failure of health professionals to comply with standards, rules, or regulations is a primary cause of such breaches. Indeed, breaches of a system's defenses and rule compliance failures are often one and the same. This chapter examines such compliance failures, especially where rules or standards of care are established, easily recognized, and widely disseminated, but professionals *consistently and even brazenly* disregard them. Worse, intentional deviations in care standards are often practiced or condoned by an entire group, such as all the nurses or technicians on a given unit. What begin as deviations from standard operating rules become, with enough repetitions, "normalized" practice patterns.[7,8] Personnel regard these acts no longer as untoward but as routine, reasonable, and entirely acceptable. These latent errors become entrenched in the system's operational architecture and dramatically enhance its vulnerability when a future active error is committed.

In this chapter I explore how stark violations of standards of practice become normalized in healthcare delivery systems, describe their motivating and enabling factors, and explain why flagrant practice deviations can persist for years. I understand "standards of care" broadly to include any standard, rule, regulation, policy, or procedure whose enactment is professionally or organizationally *required*. Because violating such standards would constitute an unreasonably unsafe act, such violations are organizationally proscribed. Consequently, the noncompliances mentioned in this chapter are dramatically different from the tweaks, improvisations, and adjustments that I discuss in chapter 2 by way of Erik Hollnagel's Safety-II paradigm. There, the practice variations are necessitated by the safety challenges of the task and in no way denote the kinds of noncompliances described in this chapter. Rather, the ones discussed here are precisely what would make Hollnagel's Safety-II experts blanch.

In this chapter, I understand "deviation" as a frank violation of an operational rule, or a variation in practice that so departs from what a rule or standard requires that an unreasonable increase in risk to patients results. Therefore, a violation of a standard or rule as illustrated in the examples below could itself be construed as a technical error.[5(p173)] Because of their chronic, seemingly benign, but frequently intentional nature, however, these rule compliance failures stand in stark contrast to one-time, unintentional, dramatic errors, like ordering the wrong medication.

This chapter concludes with a series of recommendations whereby health-care organizations might identify and manage unsafe practice deviations before they become normalized such that the interests of patient safety, quality care, and employee morale can be reliably maintained.

Deviating Practices in Healthcare

Consider the following examples of deviating practices:

1. A study recently conducted by the group VitalSmarts and the American Association of Critical Care Nurses revealed that not washing or sanitiz-ing hands sufficiently, not gowning up, skipping some other infection-control procedures, not changing gloves when appropriate, failing to check armbands, not performing safety checks, using abbreviations, not getting required approval before acting, and violating policies on stor-ing or dispensing medications are common rule-breaking practices in American hospitals.[9] Note their difference from performing a wrong-side surgery or administering a 10-fold overdose of medication to a patient.

2. A classic 2002 article by Mark R. Chassin and Elise C. Becher about a patient who was mistakenly taken for another patient and began receiving that patient's procedure noted that the subsequent investi-gation of this "wrong patient" case uncovered 17 distinct errors: "The most remediable of these were absent or misused protocols for patient identification and informed consent, systematically faulty exchange of information among caregivers, and poorly functioning teams."[10(p826)]

3. A case related to me by a physician nicely illustrates how deviations become normalized: "When I was a third-year medical student, I was ob-serving what turned into a very difficult surgery. About two hours into it and after experiencing a series of frustrations, the surgeon inadvertently touched the tip of the instrument he was using to his plastic face mask. Instead of his requesting or being offered a sterile replacement, he just froze for a few seconds while everyone else in the operating room stared at him. The surgeon then continued operating. Five minutes later he did it again and still no one did anything. I was very puzzled, but when I asked one of the nurses about it after the operation, she said, 'Oh, no big deal. We'll just load the patient with antibiotics and he'll do fine.' And, in fact, that is what happened; the patient recovered nicely."

4. A catastrophic negligence case that I participated in as an expert witness

involved an anesthesiologist who turned off a ventilator at the request of a surgeon who wanted to take an x-ray of the patient's abdomen (see Case 1.5).[11(pp87-101)] The ventilator was to be off for only a few seconds, but the anesthesiologist forgot to turn it back on (or thought he had turned it back on but had not). The patient was without oxygen for a long enough time to cause her to experience global anoxia, which plunged her into a vegetative state. She never recovered, was disconnected from artificial ventilation nine days later, and then died two days after that. It was later discovered that the anesthesia alarms and monitoring equipment in the operating room had been deliberately programmed to a "suspend indefinite" mode such that the anesthesiologist was not alerted to the ventilator problem. Tragically, the very instrumentality that was in place to prevent such a horror was disabled, possibly because the operating room staff found the constant beeping annoying.

Health professionals are hardly the only professional group to engage in or fail to attend to variations or deviations from standards or protocols. Megadisasters such as Chernobyl, Three-Mile Island, Bhopal, and the ill-fated *Challenger* and *Columbia* space missions all witnessed system flaws and protocol violations that antedated the disasters for years.[2,4,5,12] For example, the National Aeronautic and Space Administration knew about the rocket booster O-ring failures that led to the *Challenger* disaster for at least 5 years prior.[2] The debris shedding from the external fuel tank that damaged the wing of the space shuttle *Columbia*, causing the vessel to come apart 16 days later when it re-entered the Earth's atmosphere, had been a recognized design flaw for 20 years. Indeed, debris shedding had occurred on every space shuttle flight.[12] The catastrophe at Bhopal, India, where more than 2,500 people were killed and more than 200,000 injured, was preceded by six prior accidents that led to no safety improvements, a continued and heavy reliance on inexperienced operators, ignored inspector's warnings, and malfunctioning equipment.[5]

What these disasters typically show is that the factors accounting for them usually had "long incubation periods, typified by rule violations, discrepant events that accumulated unnoticed, and cultural beliefs about hazards that together prevented interventions that might have staved off harmful outcomes."[13(p294)] Especially striking is how *multiple* rule violations and lapses can coalesce to enable a disaster's occurrence, as in example 4 above. As one commentator put it, "[T]here is no isolated 'cause' of an accident. There are multiple contributors to accidents. Each of these is . . . insufficient in itself to create an accident. Indeed, it is the linking of these causes together that creates the circumstances required for the accident."[1(p2)] I now examine some reasons that practice deviations occur and how such deviations become normalized.

Factors that Account for the Normalization of Deviance

In considering the normalization of deviance, two things should be kept in mind. First, while the normalization of deviant practices in healthcare does not appear substantially different from how corrupt practices in private business evolve and become normalized, the health professional's "deviance" is almost never performed with criminal or malicious intent.[14] Second, health professionals typically justify practice deviations as being necessary or at least not opposed to accomplishing their ethically unimpeachable objective of relieving their patients' pain and suffering.[7] Nevertheless, just as the phenomena of socialization, institutionalization, and rationalization enable corrupt practices to evolve in white-collar organizations, those phenomena are similarly at work in the evolution of deviant behavior among health professionals.[14]

Institutionalization exposes newcomers to deviant behaviors, often performed by authority figures, and explains those behaviors as organizationally normative, as in example 3 above. Socialization, which is often mediated by a system of rewards and punishments, aims at determining whether the newcomer will or will not join the group by adopting the group's deviant behaviors. Rationalization enables system operators to convince themselves that their deviances are not only legitimate but acceptable and perhaps even necessary. As mutually reinforcing, institutionalization, socialization, and rationalization work to dissolve anxiety among the uninitiated by representing deviant behaviors as thoroughly rational and not immoral responses to work performance challenges.[14] I now examine some specific mechanisms—primarily instances of institutionalization and rationalization—whereby deviance becomes normalized.

"The Rules Are Stupid and Inefficient!"

This justification for violating standards might arguably be the most common. Rule or standards deviators often interpret rule compliance as irrational and a drag on productivity.[2,7,13] The deviator typically understands the problematic rule to have been handed down by authorities who appear wildly out of touch with "life in the trenches" and thus have no appreciation of the system pressures imposed on front-line care providers. Indeed, system operators might argue that perfect compliance with all the rules or standards would make it impossible to achieve productivity targets. Unsurprisingly, system operators will often invent shortcuts or workarounds when the rule, regulation, or standard seems irrational or inefficient, such as in this scenario related to me by a veteran neonatal nurse:

Case 4.1. To discourage drug diversion in a neonatal care unit, and in the days before computerized fingerprint recognition, our nurses were required to do the following when retrieving medications from the Pyxis medication cart: The nurse getting the medication would enter her password on the computer, remove the medicine from the Pyxis drawer, draw the correct amount, and administer it to the patient. If any medicine remained in the vial—which happened frequently because newborns often do not require all the medicine in the container—she was supposed to call a second nurse to the Pyxis, who would enter her password. The second entry was supposed to indicate that the second nurse observed the first nurse discarding the leftover medicine. However, because the nurses resented having to bother one another, especially when they were extremely busy with patient care measures, they simply shared their passwords with one another and entered them when they returned to the Pyxis. Not only was this an easy shortcut, but it compensated for the nurses' taking offense that administration would think them to be drug diverters. Of course it categorically defeated the purpose of the regulation.

Knowledge Is Imperfect and Uneven

System operators might not know that a particular rule or standard exists; or they might have been taught a system deviation without realizing that it was so; or they might know that a rule exists but fail to appreciate its purpose or recognize the conditions under which to implement it.[13] Confusion over standards or rules can be especially acute among professionals who feel uncomfortable asking for help or admitting ignorance in understanding and applying a standard. The problem is compounded for newly graduated professionals, who can be easy prey for learning deviant behaviors that have become normalized in their work environments. As a nurse recalled in looking back on her experience just after graduation from nursing school, "It is just the global newness . . . [I]t is kind of overwhelming. You are new to the setting, new to working, new to all the technical skills and new to the personalities. It is very difficult to hold yourself together and function in those early months. It is just kind of an overwhelming plunge, I think. Not everyone survives it."[15(pp1137-38)] Whether one is a freshly minted graduate or a seasoned professional, the introduction of new technologies and work responsibilities can easily disrupt practicing according to the recognized standard.

The Disruptive Nature of Work

Complex work environments are often dynamic, unstable, and therefore unpredictable. New technologies and personnel can disrupt ingrained practice patterns, impose new learning demands, or force system operators to devise novel responses or accommodations to new work challenges. Thus, it is still common to see computer passwords taped onto monitors in hospital units. As Richard Cook has noted, "When new technologies are used to eliminate well-understood system failures or to gain high precision performance, they often introduce new pathways to large scale, catastrophic failures. Not uncommonly, these new, rare catastrophes have even greater impact than those eliminated by the new technology."[1(p3)] Novel technologies and clinical interventions by their very nature disrupt existing knowledge and behavioral patterns and can greatly increase the probability of disaster.

"I'm Breaking the Rule for the Good of My Patient!"

This justification for rule deviation recalls the situation described in Case 4.1, where the rule or standard is understood as counterproductive. The phlebotomist in the following example might similarly plead that rule following diminished the quality of her patient care:

Case 4.2. A phlebotomist in a neonatal unit would slip on her gloves to do a blood draw but then immediately tear off the index fingertip of one of them (thus violating an infection-control rule). She would use that exposed fingertip to detect the baby's vein, which she would then stick. She claimed she had a very hard time feeling the baby's vein through the latex glove, and she didn't want to miss the vein and cause the baby to have multiple sticks. It took three rather direct confrontations with her supervisor before her rule violation stopped.[9]

"The Rules Don't Apply to Me," or "You Can Trust Me"

While pathological narcissists who believe they are above rule following can be found in many organizations, a subtler form of "the rules don't apply to me" is when system operators believe that they are not tempted to engage in the behavior that the rule or standard is supposed to deter.[11] Thus, the rule is understood as superfluous. As in Case 4.1, the rule violator feels perfectly justified in performing the problematic behavior because the deviant practice of drug diversion would never cross her mind. Administrators should appreciate a psychological finding that has been replicated in various forms throughout the twentieth century: Most human beings perceive themselves as good and decent people, such that they can understand many of their rule violations as entirely rational and ethically acceptable responses to problematic situations. They understand themselves to be doing nothing wrong and will be outraged and will often fiercely defend themselves when confronted with evidence to the contrary.[14]

Personnel Are Afraid to Speak Up

The likelihood that rule violations will become normalized obviously increases if persons who witness them refuse to intervene. Yet, a 2005 study of more than 1,700 healthcare professionals found that "it was between difficult and impossible to confront people" who manifested problematic work behaviors, especially rule breaking, incompetence, and showing disrespect.[16(p10)] Fear of retaliation, lack of ability to confront, belief that it is "not my job," and low confidence that speaking up will do any good were the chief reasons given for not calling attention to deviant behaviors. As the study reported, "People don't want to make others angry or undercut their working relationship, so they leave difficult discussions to others or to another time, and never get back to the person."[16(p10)] Obviously, human beings underlie every rule violation or system failure.[5(p201)] If personnel feel intimated or frightened to call an operator's or supervisor's attention to the deviance, it is more likely to persist and, even more problematically, to interact with other system failures, inviting disasters, as in the following example:

Case 4.3. Dr. Jackson's penmanship is frequently illegible, but he becomes very testy and sometimes downright insulting when a nurse asks him to clarify what he's written down. So rather than ask him, the annoyed nurse will proceed to the nurse's station, consult with another nurse or two, and collectively try to decipher Dr. Jackson's scrawl.

This example illustrates the linking of multiple system faults—poor handwriting that goes unremediated, resulting in nonphysicians' ordering medications that they are guessing to be correct—which someday could result in disaster.

Leadership Withholding or Diluting Findings on System Problems

Findings of system flaws and weaknesses are frequently revised and diluted as that information ascends the chain of command, for several reasons.[2,13] A supervisor might be abundantly aware of standard or rule violations but be fearful of how her unit (and, by extension, herself) would look to the administration if her superiors knew about the deviance. Marc Gerstein termed this "politics triumphing over safety," because the objective, through concealment, is to save face among one's superiors.[2(p245)] Furthermore, remediative efforts to correct standards violations might be perceived as too time consuming and as risking short-term productivity losses—such as when a hospital's misbehaving but only neurosurgeon is left to his problematic behaviors because administrators fear he will leave if confronted with his unprofessionalism.[2,17] Admittedly, the neurosurgeon's departure could be a financial blow for the hospital, from not only the lost revenues of neurosurgical procedures but the lost opportunity for neurosurgical consultations, referrals, or admissions to or from other units (e.g., neurology, oncology, or rehabilitation medicine). It is easy to understand how a hospital's administration might shrink from initiating remedial, not to mention disciplinary, measures against him.

What is as unsettling as it is interesting in these situations is how an administrator might convince herself that correcting an employee's practice deviations could be more trouble than whatever future disasters might result from those deviations. The latter are discounted as "improbable," while the former, such as the possibility of the neurosurgeon's resigning in a huff and going to a competitor hospital, are perceived as disastrous. This has led Gerstein to remark, "While safety and risk management is [sic] perfectly compatible with efficient operations over the long term, it often runs contrary to it in the short term, especially where there have been long periods of neglect. For organizations under performance pressure, getting reliable and unfiltered information through the chain of command can be all but impossible."[2(p279)]

RECOMMENDATIONS: A FUNDAMENTAL COMMITMENT TO PATIENT SAFETY

An essential sensibility in remediating the normalization of deviance begins with leadership's requiring system operators to consistently renew their commitment to patient safety.[8] Unfortunately, that commitment is as easily declared in the organization's public rhetoric as it is ignored in practice. As the famed psychologist Albert Bandura put it, "Most everyone is virtuous at the abstract level," but declarations or announcements of professionalism and patient-centered care are frequently forgotten when the idea of speaking up about system weaknesses or flawed practice behaviors arouses feelings of fear and anxiety.[18(p10)]

Over months and often years, health professionals working together can come to regard one another as members of a family in contrast to the patients they treat, who are typically admitted and discharged over a few days and whose care needs can exhaust (and often frustrate) the staff. Because of their sustained relational proximity and interdependencies, professional staff members can feel extremely supportive of or at least sympathetic toward one another. Consequently, we should not be surprised when health professionals protect one another, or at least refuse to jeopardize a team member's welfare, by keeping silent over system faults or operator errors.

But these very observations underscore the importance of periodically reminding oneself of a commitment to patient safety. Professionals must find the wherewithal to valorize duty over group self-interest, and patient safety over the personal comfort of group members.[13] A powerful way of enabling that commitment is for leadership to model it and to foster an organizational environment that eradicates, as much as possible, factors that sustain rule and standards violations. The following subsections explore how this might be accomplished.

Pay Attention to "Weak Signals"

System operators must become acutely vigilant about deviant behaviors and practices and be ready to take aggressive steps to halt their occurrence before the behaviors achieve normalization.[2] Although the above examples of deviance certainly suggest organizational problems, note that the commission of any one of them only heightens the *possibility* of injury rather than ensures it. "Heightened possibility of injury" is an abstraction, however, the normative force of which might pale in comparison to the challenge of confronting a practice deviation and correcting it. One can easily convince oneself not to intervene because a particular deviant practice has yet to result in patient harm, and the thought of intervening is unpleasant in light of the anticipated discomfort associated with confronting deviators and those who enable them.[16] On the other hand, the best time to intervene in correcting a deviant practice is early rather than later on, when righting the now normalized deviation can be much more challenging.[19]

It therefore behooves healthcare organizations to teach employees that practice deviations are common occurrences in most work environments; that deviators rarely intend harm but are probably trying to be more efficient and secure better outcomes; but that these deviations need to be identified, examined, and halted whenever they jeopardize patient care.[8] Sensitizing employees to the idea that unsafe practice deviations are not to be tolerated can occur through discussions during rounds, incident surveys and reports, and the use of focus groups. Educational activities built around root cause analyses and case studies can be useful in destigmatizing practice deviations with respect to assigning blame to individuals while simultaneously helping employees to appreciate the menacing dimensions of deviations.[12,13,19] The goal of such efforts should be to create a culture of understanding that some practice deviations are likely to occur but deserve swift attention.

Resist the Urge to Be Unreasonably Optimistic

Unfortunately, human beings can easily develop an irrational optimism about avoiding adverse events. Gerstein has discussed how persons approach practice deviations by comparing their estimation of the labor required to remediate the deviance with the probability of an adversity caused by the deviance actually occurring.[2] If the latter is perceived to be very low but the former uncomfortably high, supervisory personnel might take the easier course and convince themselves that remediating rule violations or standards deviations can be forgone. Furthermore, even though few system deviations, flaws, or weaknesses actually result in serious injury or catastrophe, that very infrequency can lull system operators into irrational complacency. In the 20 years prior to the *Columbia* space shuttle tragedy, the debris shedding that ultimately doomed the shuttle had occurred without incident on *every* previous shuttle flight.[12] As that occurrence became increasingly familiar to design engineers, its risk severity was steadily downgraded according to the illogical idea that "if no accident has happened by now, it never will."

Instead of calculating the emotional and physical toil of correcting deviances versus the probability of an accident's occurring, Gerstein suggests that one instead consider the *gravity and repercussions of an adverse event's actual occurrence*.[2] For example, even though most people have never had their homes go up in flames, few would forgo a home owner's insurance policy. That many health professionals resist making and acting on this benefits/burdens calculation even though it involves preventable harm to patients seems remarkable, which only makes the case stronger for the formidability of psychological barriers to speaking up.

Teach Employees How to Conduct Emotionally Uncomfortable Conversations *Artfully*

As noted above, confronting a system operator whose practice behaviors unjustifiably deviate from accepted standards can be extremely uncomfortable. The conversation might be marked by anger and threats from the employee that are then met with equally unproductive responses from the supervisor. Multiple authors, including Neff, Sotile and Sotile, Bernstein, and Buckman, have written valuable materials that can assist supervisors with this difficult task.[19-23] Some empathic responses that can help prevent or defuse volatile moments during such conversations are listed in box 4.1.

Some experts recommend that if the violation is not terribly serious, the first intervener should be a peer without much administrative power.[19] With physicians, peer intervention seems especially advisable. For more serious or repeat violators, a team intervention (that could include an administrator, the hospital attorney, a counselor, etc.) might be needed. In such instances, interveners must rehearse their roles, responsibilities, and communications. To believe that these activities can be breezily improvised at a meeting with a rude, hostile, and extremely defensive rule violator is thoroughly naïve. Interveners should develop and follow a script that not only outlines their dialogue, that is, what words and phrases they will actually use, but specifies the outcome they want, along with a fairly detailed plan to secure it. It is very important that after the meeting, the offending employee receive an official written summary of the discussion that outlines the next steps in the remediation. The employee should be required to acknowledge that the summary is accurate. Interveners might have to repeat this last step because the rule offender can find it distressing to acknowledge that the meeting even took place.[19]

Interestingly, administrators or supervisors tasked with these challenging conversations might be buoyed by a positive finding from the literature. Simply informing a problem employee about the unacceptability of his or her behavior has a high success/remission rate.[19] Problem employees sometimes express ignorance of their behavior or its impact. Nevertheless, perhaps the most important thing for interveners to understand is that their intervention should be prompt. The longer rule violators are left to their wayward practices, the more they will understand them as organizationally acceptable.[14]

System Operators Need to Feel Safe in Speaking Up

Assuming that leadership is committed to patient safety and to the value of speaking up, the literature recommends that organizations have policies disseminated among staff specifying instances when speaking up is expected.[16] These policies must promise protection to staff who do. Training sessions should be developed and conducted throughout the organization, largely by administrators and supervisors rather than by private consultants, on identifying and remediating system weaknesses and rule violations.[8,16,19]

Nevertheless, institutions might need to work very hard at convincing staff members that they can feel safe in speaking up or calling attention to standards or rule deviations. Fear of retaliation or the expectation of an organizational nonresponse often inhibits staff members from speaking up. Consequently, organizations might carefully consider the value of a "blameless and nonpunitive" response to errors and latent system failures.[2,11(pp132-50,24,205-13)]

Articulating a policy of blameless and nonpunitive responses to error is not without difficulties, however. For example, should all errors or practice deviations go unblamed and unpunished, even the brazenly reckless ones? Conversely, organizations that *reflexively* punish rule violators or personnel who call attention to such violations are often effectively silencing information crucial to patient safety.[2] Assuming persons who call attention to standards and rule violations are motivated by patient-centered concerns rather than selfish behaviors aimed at trying to harm fellow employees, protection must be afforded to them.[16,25] On the other hand, organizations must also treat purported rule violators fairly, as the latter might be able to justify their practice deviations or plead mitigating circumstances. For example, in determining blame for a rule violation, organizations should ask questions such as the following: (1) Was the violator properly taught or informed about the rule but chose to violate it anyway, or might the organization have failed to instruct employees adequately on the its rules, policies, and procedures? (2) Is the standard or rule routinely ignored by most organization members? If so, is the standard or rule really necessary? (3) Might a reasonable person in similar circumstances have judged a violation to be justified? (4) Were there mitigating circumstances such as sleep deprivation or malfunctioning technology that invited the practice deviation?[11,24]

These questions underscore the importance of ensuring that allegations of rule or standards violations are not only evidentially supported, but investigated from the standpoint of *the job performance pressures the system operator was experiencing when he or she engaged in the problematic behavior.*[1,3] These considerations are critical because system weaknesses, such as inadequate training or staffing, poor equipment design, or managing conflicting priorities, invite practice deviations. Still, behind every system flaw or practice deviation stands one or more human beings responsible and accountable for it, which recalls the necessity of a prompt and effective response to the rule violations and violators.

Realize that Oversight and Monitoring for Rule Compliance Are Never Ending

Richard Cook has pointed out that complex systems like healthcare are intrinsically hazardous in that they invariably contain changing mixtures of failures, weaknesses, and expertise, and they always run in a "degraded" mode.[1] A health system's defenses are never running perfectly, and technological change inevitably introduces new forms of failure.[6] Complicating this is the notion of an "acceptable" risk that seems to permeate organizational thinking. Disconcertingly, the concept of an acceptable risk implies that one is either confident enough that the system's defenses will detect, intercept, and defuse an error occurrence before its potential threat materializes, or that one has actually had prior experience with the risk materializing and deems that harm acceptable. Either rationale is worrisome. The first rests on an admittedly fallible conjecture that system defenses always work, when, as we observed in the previous anesthesia example (Case 1.5), these defenses can be short circuited. The second rationale implies a historical experience with harm-causing deviance whose next iteration might be much worse than its predecessor.[2,5,12]

Summary

This chapter shows how the commission of errors is only a piece of the mosaic of unwarranted or preventable harms. Just as important if not more so are system weaknesses or failures, which frequently appear as persistent and chronic rule violations or deviations from practice standards. In healthcare, these deviations or rule violations are rarely motivated by malice or greed; they often result from personnel feeling intense performance pressures. Amid job stress, staff can perceive rules, practice standards, and regulations as inefficient, nonsensical, counterintuitive, and even contrary to patient welfare.

Even when personnel are abundantly aware of and anxious about a colleague committing serious rule violations, they might feel inhibited about speaking up. Arguably, the psychological barriers to calling attention to deviations and deviators are the primary reason that they endure in healthcare operations.[16] Adopting a hypervigilant attitude and rapid response to practice deviations can easily give way to the comforting rationalization that "if a disaster hasn't occurred by now, it never will," along with feelings of intense discomfort triggered by the thought of taking remedial action. As such, organizations that impress on staff members that their speaking up will be valued rather than penalized are moving in a patient-centered direction.

The theme of this chapter—namely, that deviant practices in the form of violations of rules and practice standards are arch contributors to healthcare disasters—is remarkably generalizable. On March 18, 1990, the most sensational art heist in US history occurred. As reported by Stephen Kurkjian of the *Boston Globe*, a security guard at the Isabella Stewart Gardner Museum in Boston let two thieves posing as police officers into the building at 1:24 am.[26] In short order, the thieves overtook and restrained the two guards on duty, and then made off with 13 paintings and other artwork, among them three Rembrandts and a Vermeer. The value of the haul was estimated at $300–$500 million. As of this writing in 2018, none of the art has been recovered.

Post hoc analyses showed that the guard sitting at the security control desk was a then-23-year-old Berklee College of Music student. In an interview, he called the job "the most boring in the world" and confessed that he frequently arrived at work stoned on marijuana, although not on the morning in question. What he had to admit, however, was that he violated two critical rules: Never allow anyone into the Gardner after hours who hadn't been summoned by museum staff, and never leave the security desk unattended. The reason for the latter rule is that the *only* alarm switch that the Gardner had to alert police was on the security desk. Consequently, when one of the thieves lured the guard away from the desk and then handcuffed him, the museum was without its only direct contact to the Boston police. Leadership at the Gardner was well aware of this appalling security weak-

---

Box 4.1. Empathic Responses to the Problem Employee

"I'm sure you don't realize this, but . . ."

"You are very important to this organization."

"I could be wrong here."

"Can I explain what I'm seeing and get your point of view?"

"Right now, the way you do X would be considered risky or a departure from the standard of care" (focus on safety, not on competence).

"I value our friendship/relationship, and I want us to be honest with one another."

"My understanding is X; is that yours?"

"What do you think can be done about this?"

"When I bring up a concern, I see you tense up. Sometimes you cut me off or jump in with a disagreement. I think you stop listening and begin defending. You may not realize how you're coming across, but that's how it appears to me and others. Do you realize you're doing that?"[1,9,19,20,21]

---

ness; a formal recommendation to move the entire security system into a control room accessible only to those with pass keys had been submitted to the museum director the year before.[26]

Whether the disasters occur in hospitals or art museums, the contribution of protocol or rule violations that allow errors or other kinds of "toxins," like thieves, to exploit the system is confirmed time and again. System operators become careless and lackadaisical from nonevents: the last incident at the Gardner had been a botched theft that had occurred 20 years before. System operators are often untrained or inexperienced: the guards claimed that they had never been told what to do if police showed up unannounced, although the rule about refusing entry into the museum was clearly stated in the museum's security manual. And, as Richard Cook observed, systems always operate in a degraded mode: an older, more experienced guard who might have refused the thieves entry had called in sick that shift, leaving two young and inexperienced guards with one alarm switch to protect the museum's priceless artworks.[1]

Whether the prize is a Rembrandt or a patient's safety, the stakes are tremendously high. Professionals who perform rule-bound tasks, especially associated with complex and risky interventions whose failures can invite serious harm and injury, must appreciate the perils of deviating from standards of care. The more such deviations are allowed, the more normalized they become. Reminding themselves of the seriousness of the stakes might help health professionals to steel their courage, remain vigilant, and respond aggressively to unsafe practice deviations whenever they occur.

5 Humility

Never make the mistake of thinking you've made a mistake.

A surgeon to his residents, circa 1978

It is part of the human condition to suppress our inadequacies, to both ourselves and others.

Peter A. M. Anderson[1(p155)]

[H]umility . . . is perhaps the most difficult [virtue] for the contemporary physician to grapple with.

Jack Coulehan[2(p214)]

Life is suffering.

Mark Epstein[3]

Chapter Overview. This chapter begins with a historical sketch of humility, largely as it was developed by Bernard de Clairvaux. I then offer a more contemporary understanding, which seems better geared to preserving mental health and equilibrium, and segue into a discussion of humility in medicine. Here, I analyze some examples of humility's opposite, narcissism, along with commenting on the phenomenon of overconfidence, which is often thought to represent a compensatory mechanism for feelings of uncertainty that threaten one's self-esteem. The chapter ends with discussion of whether humility might be taught and how humility, or its lack, might become an object of self-awareness.

I received this chapter's first epigraph from a physician who wrote it down on a piece of paper, which he handed to me after I finished a lecture. We didn't discuss it, but I wonder how many physicians who were trained in that era would agree with it, despite its ambiguity: Did the surgeon actually recommend ignoring or paying no mind to mishaps due to mistakes, or was he suggesting that physicians learn from their outcomes and experiences but not label them as "mistakes," perhaps for fear of injuring their emotional health or inviting a lawsuit?

I begin this chapter with that quotation because if it's desirable for clinicians to develop a sense of humility, a principled resistance to admitting mistakes will not advance that cause and will likely turn out to be more troublesome than helpful. So in this chapter I discuss in considerable detail why the cultivation of humility is a good thing. By now, one reason should be crystal clear: So much of the preceding text has emphasized the need to improve thinking and cognition in heightening patient safety such that ignoring the value of learning from our limitations and our errors is a costly oversight in itself. I've heard it proposed that physicians' psychological aversion to admitting and discussing their mistakes is one reason for the lack of progress in patient safety during much of the twentieth century.

As the second and third epigraphs note, learning from and about our shortcomings is difficult. We fear that contemplating our mistakes will harm us; we discount the value of returning to our mistakes and learning what enabled or facilitated them; and like our epigraphic surgeon, we deny mistakes because we are anxious about maintaining our professional rank and self-esteem. If, through humility, we accept the Buddha's wisdom that we are immensely fallible; that our cravings for lifelong happiness and pleasure will ultimately be disappointed; and that entropy gets us all—Father Time continues to have a perfect batting average—dealing with life's manifold shortcomings and, indeed, its tragedies might become somewhat easier.

This chapter surveys humility from several perspectives. I start with a historical overview that especially focuses on the unfortunate, maladaptive ways in which humility came to be represented in the West over the last millennium. That discussion is followed by a more contemporary, empirically driven account of humility, which includes strategies for overcoming unproductive reactions to mistake and error, especially the familiar resort to overconfidence that punctuates many diagnostic errors. The chapter concludes with a discussion of strategies for improving the cultivation of humility in the twenty-first century, despite the barriers to its development in contemporary healthcare education and delivery.

A Historical Sketch

Our sketch of humility begins not with the Buddha or Jesus Christ but with Bernard de Clairvaux, the twelfth-century monastic, mystic, emissary, doctor of the Church, and political insider par excellence. Bernard was canonized a saint only twenty-one years after his death in 1153, and the various depictions of his life offer an account of an extraordinary man who, very much like a modern-day secretary of state, found himself at the center of political life and power in England and much of Europe, mediating schisms, heresies, and political upheavals both sacred and profane.[4] Perhaps chief among them were his attempts to settle the contest for the papacy between Innocent II and the antipope Anacletus II (an effort lasting eight years and ending only with Anacletus's death in 1138). He preached, taught, and wrote voluminously on the spiritual life and preparing for one's eternal reward or, more likely given Bernard's acute pessimism about the human condition, eternal damnation. He launched more than a hundred monasteries across Europe and was appointed by Pope Eugene II to inaugurate the Second Crusade (which turned into a disaster that Bernard, so some say, blamed on others).[5]

Bernard's thinking on humility became the commonly accepted account over the next 900 years. By any twenty-first-century understanding of mental health or welfare, however, Bernard's account could not be better suited to induce pathologically poor self-esteem and all the psychological ills that attend it. At the worst moments of his writings, Bernard recommends a relentless self-abasement—"becoming contemptible in your own sight"—and demands meekness, servility, obsequiousness, groveling, feelings of unworthiness, shame, silence, obedience to authority, and a reluctance to exercise one's will.[5] Of course, given Bernard's strikingly public life and his prominence as one of the great political insiders of the twelfth century, he was a host of self-contradictions. His views on humility may have been motivated by an acute anxiety—probably pressured by papal and secular demands—to put a stop to the schismatic movements occurring all over Europe. Thus and not surprisingly, Bernard's depiction of humility emphasizes an obedience to authority, perhaps as a strategic move to quiet the political and ideological unrest of his time.[6] Unfortunately, his characterization of humility is largely the one that has come down to us through the ages: as not only a self-formation or attitude marked by self-abnegation and feelings of unworthiness, but also as a mercilessly low estimation of our rank in God's creation. Indeed, some etymologists believe that "humility" may have derived from *humus*, or dirt.[7]

Some Philosophical Background

In a 1988 essay, Norvin Richards took a philosophical approach to wondering whether Bernard's thoughts on humility were logically coherent and truth consistent.[8] He noted that many if not most people are decent, law-abiding, respectable human beings whose behaviors don't fit Bernard's pessimism about humanity. But if Bernard is to be believed, are these people then to lie to themselves to preserve his opinions? Are they to say, "In truth, I'm a decent guy. I'm faithful to my wife. I work hard and honestly. I put food on the table and am loving toward my children. But according to Bernard, all of this is a deception, and I'm really a worm. No better than the dirt I walk on." Richards wonders whether such persons must then distort their seemingly accurate self-perception to accommodate Bernard's despondent view of humanity. Or is there something wrong or frankly pathological about Bernard's depiction of humility, which takes nearly rapturous satisfaction in highlighting our flaws, imperfections, and unworthiness before God? And what about the monks who tried to outdo one another in sacrifice, prayer, fasting, and other forms of self-denial? It's hard not to believe that either an intense, worldly pride was at work among them, or the relentlessly anxious preoccupation with their spiritual purity hid a false humility and modesty —a knowledge that they are or must try to be superior before their peers but which they cannot and must not admit. Furthermore, does it make for a better world when persons, especially ones who have responsibilities to others, renounce their ambitions, self-confidence, and assertiveness? Do we advance our communities and the quality of life for ourselves and others with the attitudes and behaviors Bernard advocates?[9]

Although the *Oxford English Dictionary* understands humility as "the quality of being humble or having a lowly opinion of oneself; meekness, lowliness, humbleness: the opposite of pride or haughtiness," the contemporary psychological understanding of humility recommends an entirely different brace of attributes.[7] June Price Tangney, perhaps the leading empirical researcher on humility, has offered a humility prototype, provided in box 5.1. But what I find provocative in Tangney's writings is her observation that humility is a kind of "self-forgetfulness."[10] Not only does authentic humility represent the opposite of narcissism's relentless, egocentric preoccupation, but the humble person seems relatively uninterested in his or her persona or self, that is, having no inclination to self-referentiality. This is one reason for the paucity of research on humility versus the rather large body of work on narcissism, because humble people don't particularly care to interrogate or talk about themselves. Indeed, Tangney and others have noted that humility seems antithetical to human nature's and neuroevolution's insisting that we maintain a self-focus that fosters our survival interests.[10] The truly humble person may be one of nature's rarer creatures.

Yet, it would be a mistake to think that humble people cannot be financially successful, institutional leaders, or even ambitious. The driving force, however, is not their self-aggrandizement but perhaps their pursuit of a vision of good for others or a project that invigorates them and that they believe has great social value.[11] The pathological narcissist, in contrast, cannot understand undertaking a project unless it somehow redounds to his or her glory, social standing, or wealth. And because many narcissists like to boast about their accomplishments, they tend to be tiresome and off-putting; it is abundantly obvious that these people will be decidedly disinterested in the welfare of others when their own self-interests are at stake.[12]

An obvious question that the research literature has not resolved is whether humble people are born rather than made. A good deal of anecdotal observation relates how certain people's personalities have gone from selfish to humble after a tragic or unsettling life event impressed them with life's tentativeness, finitude, unpredictability, nastiness, and occasional compassion and generosity.[13] These transformative events tend to be *limbic* experiences, because to don the cloak of humility, our neurocircuitry might need a dramatic overhaul somewhat like a religious conversion. But why would one want to effect that conversion, assuming choice enters the picture? Not only are the benefits of humility nonobvious, but we associate humility with a character type that seems boring and defeatist. Why would one want to do it or even be interested? Convincing someone to practice the strategies of humility or to embrace a humble perspective on the world can be a difficult sell.

The Benefits of Humility

Perhaps the outstanding benefit of humility is its engendering what psychologists call excellent self-calibration, which is marked by an absent need to distort information in a self-inflating way—something to which narcissists are particularly prone.[10] The humble person's psychological defenses are nowhere near the stratospheric levels of the calcified narcissist, who is devastated by failure and anxiously looks to blame others when serious adversity from error or misjudgment strikes. Whereas some narcissistic types are keenly vulnerable to shame and are inclined to think of themselves as better than they really are—a trait also shared with much of humanity in general—the humble person is somehow without this need or attitude.[14] Humble persons instead tend to minimize their sense of self (and thus are less vulnerable to self-disesteeming experiences), but they will readily admit their imperfections and flaws. Indeed, it is thought that a "healthily" humble attitude assists an individual in securing a clearer, more objective view of his or her own and others' performance, such that strengths and weaknesses are more obvious, and corrective strategies and remedies are less resisted (or better welcomed) because they are not experienced as humiliating or shameful.[15]

Some scholars have opined that improving the practice of the virtues begins with strengthening or deepening our humility, perhaps because humility might enable a clearer understanding of our intentions, motivations, and limitations.[16] Arijit Chatterjee and Donald C. Hambrick wrote an interesting paper in 2007 in which they argued that narcissistic chief executive officers of large corporations—whose narcissism was represented by self-referential statements like their use of the word "I" in public announcements, the number of times they authorized photographs of themselves in their company's marketing and media materials, and their readiness to appear on media or issue media statements—exposed their companies to topsy-turvy fluctuations in earnings and acquisitions much more often than their non-narcissistic counterparts.[17] The authors speculated that narcissistic leaders enjoy the attention and admiration that accompanies significant risk taking, especially when they can take credit for successes and blame others for failures. But their irrepressible penchant for the spectacular makes for a wild corporate ride, which the authors believe is usually no more or less successful than the business trajectory of more cautious and restrained leaders. Recent research on more humble leaders indicates that they tend to shape their managerial styles according to a shared vision of their organization's mission and performance goals, as in a "we're in this together" philosophy. Humble leaders perceive the strengths of others and share power with them, and their leadership teams report feeling highly committed toward their organization's mission and performance goals.[18]

The primary interest of this chapter, however, is to examine the role of humility in the formation of healthcare decisions and practices. I begin by considering some examples of humility failures; proceed to the challenges of "teaching" humility to medical students and future clinicians; and conclude with recommendations for implementing humility-like strategies in healthcare delivery.

Humility and the Practice of Medicine

Three particular instances of humility merit our consideration. I am indebted to a former student for this first one:

Case 5.1. The patient was a middle-aged male who appeared in the emergency room complaining of chest pain. His EKG showed ST elevations of an ongoing heart attack with positive enzymes. The patient was promptly taken to the cath lab for an emergency catheterization. The cardiologist determined, however, that the patient's heart disease was too advanced for angioplasty or stent placement and contacted Dr. Moore, the heart surgeon on call, to perform a triple bypass.

Dr. Moore had a reputation at the hospital for the unusual quickness with which he performed surgeries. His skills were regarded as average, however, and there were anecdotal reports that one reason for his speed was that he occasionally did only the minimum surgery necessary. For instance, if a patient needed three bypasses but also had two other small vessels with blockages that were borderline operative (~60 percent blocked), Dr. Moore might not operate on the small vessels even though doing so would relieve the patient's angina.

Returning to this case, Dr. Moore trusted the cardiologist's judgment and, without seeing the patient, phoned the hospital operator to page the open heart team on call to come in for an emergency coronary artery bypass graft (CABG). These preparations began at approximately 7 pm. The patient, team, and operating room were ready about an hour later. In the meantime, the anesthesiologist performed a transesophageal echocardiogram and determined that the patient had severe mitral regurgitation that needed repair.

Dr. Moore walked into the operating room thinking he was doing only a triple bypass, which would take 2.5 to 3.5 hours. When the anesthesiologist told Moore that the patient would additionally need a mitral valve repair because of the regurgitation, Moore was adamant that he was only going to do the CABGs. The anesthesiologist responded that the patient's mitral regurgitation was severe, but it looked like it could be repaired with a simple annuloplasty ring. The repair would add another hour to the surgery, however. Moore responded with an angry "Screw the MR! He's going home with it." As the surgery progressed, Moore remarked that after revascularization with the bypasses, the MR would improve. The team believed that this was true only among patients with mild MR, while this patient's was severe. After the procedure was over, team members felt terribly downcast, as they believed that within two years the patient would need a high-risk operation to repair his diseased mitral valve.

Dr. Moore might argue that adding another hour to the procedure would have created a significant morbidity risk for this patient's damaged heart. But the team believed that most other surgeons would have repaired the valve. Alas, rather than report Dr. Moore, the team did nothing. The patient was eventually discharged, leaving his condition to the next surgeon to deal with.

Case 5.2. Some years ago, I traveled to a distant state to give an invited talk. The night before my talk, I was taken out to dinner by the physician organizers of the conference. As doctors sometimes do, they began talking about their colleagues. I particularly remember this piece of conversation, which over the course of my career, I've heard in various forms multiple times. Consider the physicians jumping in and out of their cross-talk:

"So, how about Dr. Magnificent?"

"Oh God, he's a wizard."

"Yeah, amazing. So thorough and precise."

"Totally. A tightly wound guy, but a surgeon's surgeon."

"You know, he doesn't strike me as being very happy. And he's been sued four or five times."

"Well, his personality gets in the way. I've seen him being rude and arrogant, and he's very awkward at talking to patients and families when things don't go well."

"And I've seen him throw his colleagues under the bus. There's a story about him and an anesthesiologist going out to talk to a family after a surgery that didn't go well. Magnificent is nervous and doing all the talking while the anesthesiologist just stands there. And Magnificent starts by saying, 'As soon as we induced the anesthesia, things went downhill.' The anesthesiologist nearly peed his pants."

"There's another story about him walking down a hallway, seeing a family at the other end, and turning around and walking the other way."

"We've all been there." (Laughter)

"Helluva surgeon, though."

"Yeah."

Case 5.3. The following case was described at a patient safety conference in Canada by James Reason. I may have some details wrong, but the gist of the story is preserved:

A cardiothoracic resident surgeon was performing a complex surgery with the attending surgeon standing alongside, intently watching and advising. At a critical point in the surgery, the resident accidentally nicked an adjacent structure and just froze. The attending surgeon realized what had happened and gently stepped in and began to repair the nick. He said to the resident, "You know, in a way, I'm glad you did that because I can show you how to fix it."

If the psychological continuum from narcissism to humility involves one's sense of social status, power, and security, something like that seems clearly at work in Case 5.1, in which the surgeon's apparent need to exercise control and feel a sense of self-protectedness results in the patient's being left poorly off. We can only wonder what kinds of feelings and motivations allowed this surgeon to leave the patient with serious morbidity that could have been fixed. The surgeon probably feels confident that the patient's mitral regurgitation will improve, but what is damning in this case is how the surgeon's prioritizing his own agenda over the patient's may have distorted his appreciation of the patient's condition and the long-term outcome of the surgery. If the surgeon thought that adding another hour to an already three- to four-hour surgery was too much to bear, would it not have been better to admit that and secure another surgeon's help than to forgo the mitral valve repair? But the failure to confess his limitations, his arrogant insistence on being in control at the cost of an ethically deplorable decision, and the unchecked rationalization of his judgment (and refusing to notice the dejection of the staff) made for something of a tragedy. Perhaps, too, the surgeon was feeling sorry for himself having to do a lengthy procedure at night and channeled his anger into a stubborn insistence on his authority.

If humility improves our perceptions of others' needs and feelings as well as of our own limitations and imperfections, this surgeon could have been mightily assisted by a strong dose of it. Indeed, one shudders to think of how many stories there are like this one and how many patients could have fared better if their physicians had managed their anxieties by requesting help and support rather than incorporating work-around strategies or doing a halfway job.

Assuming we know nothing else about Dr. Magnificent in Case 5.2, an analysis of his behavior and professional formation might go like this: Maarit Johnson and Geoffrey R. Patching have claimed that "competence may enhance a good sense of self-esteem but contribute little if basic self-esteem is impoverished . . . [S]uccess and competence are unlikely to improve an individual's self-esteem if the perception of one's own deed is over-critical due to an impoverished basic self-acceptance."[16(pp44,46)] One would be hard pressed not to think that self-esteem anxieties are at the core of Dr. Magnificent's personality. Typically, and all the professions have many of them, these individuals concentrate on transcendent skill development, acquiring immense (but somehow never enough) professional prestige and collecting as many external markers of success as they can to soothe their self-esteem anxieties.[19] Psychologists would say they are "anxious about their lovability."[20] They have learned and internalized the idea, often at an early age, that they can calm that anxiety and compensate for their low self-estimation with a relentless quest for mastering skills that matter to them and bring them praise. Mediocrity is exactly what their low self-esteem cannot tolerate, since it confirms what they most fear: that they are only average and "therefore" worthless. Not surprisingly, Dr. Magnificent dedicates himself to a life of hard work, and perhaps taking advantage of a significant dose of natural talent, he finds a way to placate his mostly unconscious but ever-present need to feel positive about himself. Deep down, people like Dr. Magnificent have never acquired and internalized those psychological structures that would enable them to be at ease with themselves without the external trappings of professional success and admiration from others.[21]

Much psychological theory, especially of previous decades, places the blame with the parents' failure to convey sentiments of lovability to the child that he or she then internalizes.[22] Having "failed" at being lovable, narcissistic people resort to soothing their anxious egos with a substitute, namely, whatever they learn will attract attention and respect from significant others, such as becoming a star athlete, stellar student, beauty queen, or whatever they understand will garner expressions of social worth and respect. The core problem, however, is that their lovability insecurities never go away. Dr. Magnificent remains the prickly personality who is always anxious about the next situation that threatens his sense of self. Despite his vocation as a healer, his psychological tolerance of human suffering is thin, such that he can spend 10 hours in surgery but cannot spend 3 minutes with an upset family. Dr. Magnificent's investment in technical perfection has invited a relentless and pitiless task master into his life who doesn't miss a thing. Indeed, if Dr. Magnificent has brittle or malignant self-esteem, he may easily develop sadomasochistic tendencies as a result of the psychological machinations he uses to maintain his (easily damaged) self-regard.[23] The upset or unhappy family who project their disappointment onto Dr. Magnificent will dredge up the failures, disapprovals, and rejections that he consciously and unconsciously works to suppress, deny, or, most of all, defend against. No wonder he walks the other way when he sees disappointed or complaining family members approaching. Of course, he knows that perfection or superlative performance is unattainable in every case, but he finds ways to deny (or rationalize or dismiss) his failures because they are so painful. Yet, and rather tragically, his self-esteem anxieties are always poking through his narcissistically based defenses, which can make Dr. Magnificent an unhappy man who is probably hard to live with. Because humility is a thoroughly foreign notion to him, he cannot take advantage of its healing and restorative power, as can the resident surgeon in Case 5.3.

I love to relate Case 5.3 in lectures even though I've gotten criticized over the "I'm glad you did this" part, which sounds like the patient's welfare is subordinate to the importance of the resident's learning experience. So, I tend to deflect that criticism by turning my attention to the attending surgeon's realism and humility.

One of the great benefits of humility is what Jack Coulehan called an "unpretentious openness," which he understands as an awareness of one's own deficiencies and acceptance of the possibility that there might be other and better decisions and techniques available.[2] Other scholars have discussed the humble person's excellent self-calibration, meaning accurate insight into one's skill set and the strengths and weaknesses of others.[15] The humble person is somehow free of the way narcissism distorts self-estimation by persuading the individual that he or she is a significant cut above the rest. The humble person does not succumb to narcissistic pathologies, such as feeling extreme envy over the successes of others and being quick to blame others when things go wrong. Also, the narcissist who is embarrassed or humiliated by another never forgets it.[10]

The reality of Case 5.3 is that surgical nicks to adjacent anatomical structures do happen and in some instances are virtually unavoidable. The attending surgeon's realistic acceptance of that may explain his refraining from blaming his resident—something Dr. Magnificent would not only likely do but also lace his blame with humiliating pronouncements to "teach" the resident how a "real" surgeon is supposed to react to such an incident. The attending surgeon of Case 5.3, however, disabuses himself of all that and instead seizes the opportunity to teach his resident how to recover from an adversity. James Reason has famously said that the primary difference between experts and amateurs is that experts know how to prevent an error or mistake from turning into a calamity, which amateurs and neophytes have yet to learn.[24] The expert is not necessarily more brilliant than the learner, but he or she is more experienced and equipped to handle the unfamiliar and unexpected.

June Tangney has also noted how humility inhibits anger and can foster forgiveness.[10] If true, the reason may be that anger is often a reaction to our failing to control some situation that is going in an upsettingly different direction than the one we want. Anger may well represent our neural circuits registering (1) a realization that the world is not going as we need and want it to go, such that (2) our social rank and sense of self-esteem are painfully threatened, resulting in (3) a very anxious feeling, registered by an affective outburst, to regain control and mastery of the situation (which anger often accomplishes). One hopes that the resident absorbs the lesson that things can and will go wrong in surgery—and whether the resident's inadvertent nick should count as an error is difficult if not impossible to know—and that the mature response is to be prepared with recovery strategies so that the adversity doesn't worsen. Norvin Richards has remarked that dignity is a sense of "self-honoring," and one would like to think that the resident and the attending surgeon dignified their relationship by the way forgiveness and tolerance turned a mishap into a benefit in the learner's life (and, one hopes, without the patient's suffering adversity).[8(p317)]

The Problem of Overconfidence

What would Bernard de Clairvaux think of all this? I suspect he would be very upset over how the above is situated in a philosophically secular world, which dismisses his theological narrative of human life playing out in a divinely sanctioned order, where only faith, humility, good works, and the sacraments will save our souls. Instead, our secular account of humility concentrates on the connections among emotional health, a realistic appraisal of human performance and its limitations, and a deep appreciation of our knowledge constraints. Once again, I recall Herbert Simon's notion of "bounded rationality," which the humble person would readily embrace: namely, that humans are irrevocably beset by cognitive limitations and imperfections; that the information we have to understand and navigate our worlds is invariably degraded in terms of its accuracy, sufficiency, relevance, and so on; and that our cognitive performance is often contaminated by ecological pathogens or production pressures.[25] We do not care to admit, much less contemplate, any of this for reasons already enumerated. But what we have not yet examined is a common defensive reaction to bounded rationality, and how it occurs especially in medicine: overconfidence.

Whereas Coulton made the marvelous observation that the best antidote for hubris is to develop a sense of irony, a rather large literature has discussed a more problematic but more common alternative.[26] The experience of uncertainty, especially in high-stakes endeavors like healthcare, can be very upsetting. It leaves one feeling paralyzed, incapacitated, and unable to move forward.[27] It interferes with prognosticating outcomes, which, in turn, compromises planning a course of treatment. Worst, it provokes painful feelings of inadequacy and helplessness, especially among professionals who think they should always have the right answer to any question they are asked and should always be able to chart a patient's clinical course with unerring assurance. Yet, although we know that diagnostic accuracy is inversely proportional to the complexity of a case, we have also learned that diagnostic confidence increases proportionally with the case's difficulty.[28]

That finding should concern us, because confidence should increase with clinical accuracy rather than diagnostic complexity. If feelings of confidence (or a lack of confidence) are the brain's way of registering its cognitive accuracy, then overconfidence increasingly looks like a misestimation—it encourages the belief that one's accuracy is better than it really is.[29] Thus, as Eta Berner and Mark Graber have remarked, overconfidence represents a mismatch between perceived and actual performance.[30] They reported that physicians who were least expert or who had the lowest skill levels tended to be most confident about their judgment or performance. Just as gamblers become increasingly confident about their bets *after* they've placed them, so many clinicians are thought to use overconfidence as a way of assuring themselves of their adequacy and soothing their feelings of uncertainty.[31] Apparently, overconfidence works so well in diluting self-esteem threats that it will often dissuade the clinician from requesting second opinions, curbside consultations, or reference materials: "Overconfidence results at times from a desire to see the self as a competent or accurate perceiver. According to this perspective, undue confidence often arises when uncertainty would challenge valued beliefs about the self as knowledgeable and competent."[28,31(p373)]

In chapter 7, I discuss a case in which an infant's clinicians demurred on ordering a bilirubin test that would have detected his jaundice and possibly prevented his lifelong disabilities. The haunting question in cases like these is, Was there insufficient evidence to recommend the test such that, though the delay had tragic consequences, it was nevertheless clinically justifiable? Or was the evidence for ordering the bilirubin test reasonably compelling, but the clinicians' unjustified degree of confidence interfered with their doing so?

The phenomenon of overconfidence returns us to Croskerry's insistence on teaching debiasing strategies, because situations that provoke feelings of uncertainty can easily provoke clinicians to seek the comfort of over-confidence.[32] Feelings of robust but possibly unwarranted confidence will prompt their belief that they are on the right diagnostic path and relieve them of the weariness of pursuing System 2 methods, which require them to interrogate their thinking and impression formation. The worry is that in pursuing the relief that overconfidence provides, clinicians may fall prey to various cognitive biases, especially anchoring and confirmation biases, and only look for evidence that confirms their decisions, which may well have happened in the jaundice case.[32]

What do these observations entail? At least two interrelated remedies, the first of which is to lower the threat of admitting ignorance or uncer-tainty.[31] The second is more general: accept and internalize the truth of bounded rationality and develop epistemic aids that improve the reliability of clinical reasoning. The more hubristically or narcissistically inclined cli-nician is likely to be unenthusiastic, even uncomprehending, toward either one; the humble clinician would likely welcome both with resigned but open arms.

On Being Humble in Healthcare

To recap what we have so far: Hubristic clinicians will resist System 2 meth-ods of mindfulness in moments of uncertainty because they perceive them as tiresome and unnecessary. These individuals will be more inclined to fol-low their "instincts," which, unfortunately, are distorted by their need to feel confident if not magnificent. Those distortions will in turn result in a resis-tance to admitting uncertainty and, hence, a refusal to use epistemic supports that can assist in diagnostically complex cases. The unfortunate result is that some patients will go for long periods without the diagnostic workups they should have; a nasty disease or ailment, which will not self-resolve, will unnecessarily go untreated; symptoms won't resolve, which will cause pa-tients psychological suffering in addition to their symptomatic discomforts;

and a lawsuit for a missed, wrong, or delayed diagnosis becomes a real possibility.[33]

Humble practitioners, however, not only recognize their cognitive imperfections but admit them and disallow them from wounding their sense of self. Humble people aren't flippant or casual about their errors; but they will resist blaming others and resorting to denials or rationalizations that would otherwise protect their sense of self.[10] Nevertheless, if we examine the psychological and ethical formation of health professionals, it seems safe to say that humility is hardly an item on everyone's lips; that its lessons have never been widely integrated into healthcare curricula; that defensive behaviors arising from self-esteem threats from errors or poor outcomes are much more common than demonstrations of humility; and that an empathic but unflinchingly honest disclosure of error to patients and their families continues to be extremely challenging at many hospitals. So, why is that?

Humility enthusiasts (if such types exist) often cite physician Jack Coulehan's observations on humility in his 2011 essay "A Gentle and Humane Temper." The essay is notable not only for the depth of Coulehan's insights but also for his dismay over the "faint praise" humility receives in the curriculum as well as in practice. Here is one of Coulehan's juiciest passages:

> [N]owadays, humility is hardly a valued ideal. The words "good physician" call upon an image of confidence, technical skill, and assertiveness, a cluster of characteristics that seem inconsistent with humility . . . [H]umility appears weak, wishy-washy, counterproductive, or even deceptive . . . Few students in 2011 conceive of their education in terms of character formation at all, let alone see humility as part of it. Does anyone still believe that virtue is its own reward? . . . Imagine, if you will, a full-page spread in the *New York Times* headlined with the words: OUR DOCTORS RANK AMONG THE MOST HUMBLE IN THE UNITED STATES. WE ADMIT OUR MISTAKES. WE READILY ACKNOWLEDGE OUR LIMITATIONS.[2(p207,214)]

These words nicely capture one reason that we have done poorly with managing harm-causing errors, admitting their frequency and learning from them, and teaching the next generation of health professionals about cognitive traps and pitfalls to mitigate their threat and impact. Many professional egos simply won't allow it, while professionals of any ilk are easily thrown off-kilter at the suggestion that they may have erred. So, they typically scurry about to find face-saving strategies that deflect the ego threat.

Of course, they may equally fear being fired or sued, but most errors are not career menacing.[34]

The literature suggests numerous reasons that humans have an overall aversion to admitting their errors and to regarding them as valuable learning tools. Quite possibly, the need to feel competent and adequate, to believe in oneself, to feel confident sometimes to the point of arrogance are evolutionarily adaptive. I would argue that because humans are social animals, we feel an enduring need to always appear competent and reliable to our group members, such that we will resist a frank admission of our flaws and foibles because doing so threatens our group membership.[35]

In healthcare training, a resistance to contemplating error and learning the kinds of lessons humility can teach may also be culturally ingrained. First, students who are admitted to healthcare training institutions have not succeeded by making numerous errors and mistakes during their high school and undergraduate years. Because admission to medical or nursing school is predicated on stellar academic performance, many of these students likely have a marked aversion to making mistakes, viewing cognitive error as the enemy of their career aspirations. Moreover, as Christopher Peterson and Martin Seligman have noted, children who grew up in parental environments that (1) placed an extreme emphasis on performance, (2) routinely compared the children with others in assessing their "worth," and (3) communicated to the children their comparative superiority or inferiority in a way that was peppered with excessive praise or blame are likely to turn those children into intensely competitive, self-preoccupied individuals who may have trouble in later life accepting themselves as they are.[15] Ironically, though, that kind of emotional and maturational home environment will often produce extremely high-functioning performers, because they are forever anxious about succeeding or winning and will work very hard to maintain their identity as superbly competent. Unfortunately, many of these kinds of persons may find themselves depressed, frustrated, and angry later in life when the external trappings of success fail to bring them the happiness they were primed to expect.[3]

Second, because the stakes of caring for sick patients in complex work environments are so high, these students' professors and supervisors may have developed their own aversion to mistake making. The surgeon who was forgiving and humble in the face of his resident's nicking an adjacent anatomical structure, seizing it as a learning opportunity, may therefore be quite unusual. In any case, how twentieth-century healthcare instructors could become incensed over their students' errors is easy to under-stand since errors might not only seriously harm patients but also reflect unfavorably on the institution's judgment in admitting the student into its program as well as on the quality of training being provided. A generation ago, physician instructors were often said to "teach" by way of humilia-tion and embarrassment, while nursing instructors were said "to eat their young."[36]

Third, as Coulehan pointed out, the healthcare industry, largely through its silence, has coddled a public into thinking that its professionals don't commit errors and that healthcare environments are perfectly safe. Today's public would likely be appalled by Coulehan's imagined *New York Times* headline lauding the humility of a hospital's doctor group readily admit-ting to mistakes. But that only underscores how our expectations have been shaped by a well-intentioned but sometimes dishonest healthcare es-tablishment that is quick to announce its successes but equally quick to bury its embarrassments. If various patients' rights initiatives and patient safety groups had not been insistent about the need to improve safety in our nation's hospitals, I think it doubtful that today's institutions would have reached their current levels of transparency and safety.

Can Humility Be Taught?

If professionals, not only in healthcare but everywhere, have deep-seated reservations about admitting error but simultaneously acknowledge that they cannot truthfully deny error occurrences nor the importance of con-taining if not eliminating their causes, then at least we can expose health-care students to patient safety theory and the psychological challenges in providing care. A special challenge will be the self-attribution bias, through which people tend to take credit for their successes but blame others for their failures—related to how humans tend to accentuate the positives of their performance and ignore, deny, or deflect the negatives.[10] Every rotation or practicum that healthcare students experience should include highly de-tailed descriptions of where things can go wrong and what prevention strat-egies exist to reduce the likelihood of adversity occurrence. And it would be best for students to hear these accounts from experienced and respected faculty, who are willing to don the cloak of humility and disabuse students of the idea that mistakes and errors are perpetrated only by the inexperi-enced, the uninformed, and the inept. This will mean, of course, that fac-ulty have the backbone to engage in such self-scrutiny, are committed to the value of transparency in teaching patient safety, and won't fear looking imperfect in their self-revelations.[37]

Indeed, if professionals are going to progress toward humility, that progress seems to require considerable self-awareness and scrutiny. As such, students and professionals should be encouraged to gain greater insight into themselves, especially about their anxieties, fears, and, as someone pointed out to me, hatreds, because you can learn a lot about a person according to what he or she hates. Small group discussions led by an experienced facilitator may be the best way of proceeding, but the goal will be to overcome those inhibitions that prevent students from appreciating their performance and cognitive limitations. Included in this learning should be an exploration of suffering as it is witnessed in patient care and as life's inevitably entropic course affects us all. Learning should especially include how patients will project their suffering onto their treating professionals, or "share" it with them, and how the professional must be able to deploy self-regulatory but also therapeutic techniques when that happens.[38] Importantly, humility is thought to confer a therapeutic advantage to those who witness and tend to another's suffering, as the humble person entertains no false fantasies that he or she will be spared it, but accepts the reality of suffering as one of life's inevitabilities.

Humility might also dispose the clinician toward a more empathic, other-oriented sensibility, because "Humility is not thinking less of yourself. It is thinking of yourself less," a statement frequently attributed to C. S. Lewis but now ascribed to Rick Warren, author of *The Purpose Driven Life*.[39] The narcissist is hard pressed to do this as his or her relentless self-preoccupation is constantly interfering with an empathic effort to understand or imagine another's experience, to walk in that person's shoes.

Teamwork and Group Work as Humility Learning

Various facets of hospital or clinic teamwork could serve as excellent humility-building platforms.[40] Most humans live and work alongside others and depend on mutual cooperation and complex interdependencies to succeed. Group members come to know one another if not intimately, then at least well enough to be acquainted with their co-workers' abilities, strengths, limitations, interests, proclivities, and faults. And, as a colleague pointed out to me years ago, the best thinking is often done in groups, especially when it comes to resolving problems that arise from complex social interactions involving multiple contrasting problem sets, such as economic, psycholog-

ical, social, legal, scientific, technological, and clinical, and whose integration no single individual could master. Furthermore, everyone wants to appear competent and valuable to other group members, which can be both a
boon and a bane: a boon because with others, we learn social competency
skills and hence have a ready opportunity to test those skills, but a bane in
that social hierarchies often *discourage* members' confronting and correcting one another's problematic behaviors, such that poor performance can
easily go uncorrected and prevent the social network from advancing.[41]

Think of how effective teamwork can "optimally calibrate" the performance of team members: They can implement simulation training and
mentoring where learners (and even experts, who can always learn something new) can create or explore new knowledge, ideas, and skills. Team
member interactions can focus on developing good communication skills;
improving decision making; learning from one another's mistakes; revisit-
ing and examining the architecture of botched cases; developing epistemic
and organizational strategies that will prevent future error or disaster occurrences; and taking advantage of the supreme feedback mechanism that
teams enjoy, namely, to understand and see oneself as others do.[42]

But all this can be very threatening for the narcissistically inclined such
that they might embrace teamwork skills only if they identify themselves
as leaders. Effective teamwork interactions are antithetical to persons with
narcissistic leanings because anything suggesting equality (as among team
members) runs contrary to the narcissist's need to feel superior. Recall
Dr. Magnificent. He cannot abide anything that reminds him of his flaws or
failures. Almost to a certainty, he will resist the feedback, shared decision
making, and other-generated correctives that teamwork can offer, as he is
only comfortable within the recesses of his interiority, where his psychological defenses will work hard to protect his sense of self from the assaults
of the external world.

Conclusion

An enormous problem that stands in the way of instilling humility is that
so many high-performing professionals got that way by learning to avoid
errors early in their lives and then figured out strategies that would either
eliminate errors or dilute the error's negative effects on their goals or careers. If such persons' aims have been to eliminate errors from their performance as a key strategy toward securing their vocational aspirations, then
a medical school or residency program's claims that it will better tolerate

mistakes will seem strikingly odd. Indeed, such persons may well be bewildered by it because they are unfamiliar with environments that tolerate mistakes, lower the importance of feeling knowledgeable, and decrease the threat inherent in admitting ignorance. And yet, progressive teaching institutions should try to implement such a learning environment because learning from error is one of the most valuable pedagogical tools we have.

Still, we continue to struggle with developing reasonably safe environments because the seeming insurmountability of the challenge has largely resulted from neuroevolutionary adaptation falling short. In other words, neuroevolution has simply not caught up with twenty-first-century cognitive demands imposed by the social, economic, and technological dimensions of our environments. Climate change is a superb example: The carbon fuel industry has witnessed remarkable technological and economic development over the last two centuries and has enabled a way of life that people living in industrially advanced societies will not surrender. But the best scientific evidence indicates that unless we substantially curb carbon emissions, we will invite global catastrophe. Yet, many persons deny that prognosis and refuse to make any significant sacrifices that will make the planet safer for future generations, largely because they will not give up the comforts that are connected with carbon emissions.

System 1 and 2 reasoning modalities provide excellent examples of our neuroevolutionary shortcomings, as System 1 responses are marvelously attuned to our making rapid safety calculations and launching usually successful behavioral outputs. Interestingly, precisely that same mechanism gets Dr. Smith in trouble when she is pressured to come up with a diagnosis but lacks the relevant clinical knowledge inputs as well as the time to upgrade her understanding and thinking (such as by consulting with a colleague or studying some literature on her patient's symptoms). Furthermore, while she might be thoroughly unaware of her epistemic shortcomings, she is intensely aware of her organization's production quotas, such that she easily succumbs to an occasional half-baked diagnosis that she can only hope is right. She manages her feelings of uncertainty with an unjustified degree of confidence, however, and she communicates her therapeutic optimism to her patient, whose own System 1 network resists being critical of her decision making. Note that this is not unlike the behavior we witness from many persons who deny the threat of global warming, smoke cigarettes, ignore their being dangerously overweight, and refuse to curb their risky behaviors. Their Cro-Magnon neurocircuitry continues to favor maximizing self-interest in ways that soothe their survival anxieties, resulting in subordinating or dismissing concerns over a society's long-term economic and bioecological well-being.

Unless we overcome our inertia and do the difficult work that System 2 reasoning demands, it seems only a matter of time before we witness unprecedented harm to human life. While our socioeconomic problems are legion, the primary problem that faces contemporary healthcare professionals is their achieving an ethically judicious control of the deployment of current and near future medical technology. By all accounts, that technology will result in unprecedented costs to our national budgets—whether in the form of the latest generation of treatments for cancer or new drugs and devices that will increase longevity for the exploding numbers of older citizens and, especially, the very old. The national resistance to taking decisive but painful steps to relieve these and many more problems is remarkable.

If Croskerry is right that "the first step is to overcome the bias against overcoming bias," then I would like to think that humility is one of the most important virtues our citizenry and its government should cultivate.[43(p776)] Doing so might accelerate the adaptational process in ways that natural selection can't. The hope for superior self-calibration might especially involve the one thing that the electorate of a liberal democracy cannot be without, namely, sound critical thinking. If humility confers an advantage in cognitive accuracy and liberates people from their arrogance, egocentrism, and unscientific thinking, it may better help us manage the intersection of human limitations with the relentless onslaught of new social problems. What a national sense of humility could accomplish is to foster our collective decision making—whether about patient safety or foreign or domestic challenges—according to the best evidence or data we have, rather than according to some factually unreliable but feel-good remedy that appeases our System 1 needs for comfort and reassurance.[44]

The cultivation of humility is thought to make the cultivation of other human virtues easier. Certainly in matters of patient safety, that sounds right. If the prominent virtues of patient safety include vigilance, mindfulness, and compliance, then humility might be the foundational virtue that equips clinicians to practice the others more reliably and consistently. While the Dr. Magnificents of the world may always be vulnerable to self-esteem assaults, and use arrogance, condescension, and distancing as psychological defenses, the primary challenge of delivering healthcare for many clinicians is that it is psychologically, physically, and cognitively draining. Their

Box 5.1. Humility Traits

- Open to new paradigms
- Eager to learn from others
- Acknowledges limitations and seeks to learn from them
- Accepts failure without undue emotional burden
- Performs accurate self-appraisal
- Seeks advice
- Develops and respects others
- Desires to serve
- Shares honors and recognition
- Accepts success with restraint
- Resists adulation
- Resists self-preoccupation
- Practices restraint or self-effacement
- Does not feel special
- Appreciates the value of all things
- Practices modesty[2,17,45]

workloads are oppressive; they continually cope with technologically complex systems that don't run reliably; and they have to manage with information shortfalls, lack of resources, and fallible and occasionally unreliable colleagues. The blessing of humility is to eliminate the need to appear faultless or supremely competent and to accept the fact that, as Croskerry noted, "We all face a lifetime of vulnerability."[42(p721)] A collective acceptance of the value of humility seems an immensely healthy undertaking. Every generation should insist on instilling such a realization, which, if the musings of this book are correct, should be manifest in error reduction and a safer healthcare system. Paradoxically, we need to develop a greater tolerance for serious error, at least in the sense that when it appears, we will receive it without anger or looking to blame. Humility can teach us to do that. We should therefore avail ourselves of its lessons.

Interview with June Price Tangney

June Price Tangney received her PhD in clinical psychology from UCLA and is currently university professor and professor of psychology at George Mason University in Fairfax, Virginia. She is a recipient of the International Society for Self and Identity's Distinguished Lifetime Career Award as well as George Mason University's Teaching Excellence Award. She is also a fellow of the Association of Psychological Science and of the American Psychological Association's Division of Personality and Social Psychology. Professor Tangney is coauthor with Ronda Dearing of *Shame and Guilt*, coeditor with Ronda Dearing of *Shame in the Therapy Hour*, coeditor with Jess Tracy and Richard Robins of *The Self-Conscious Emotions: Theory and Research*, and coeditor with Mark Leary of the *Handbook of Self and Identity*. She has served as associate editor for the *American Psychologist* and *Self and Identity* and as consulting editor for the *Journal of Personality and Social Psychology, Personality and Social Psychology Bulletin, Psychological Assessment, Journal of Social and Clinical Psychology*, and *Journal of Personality*. Her research on the development and implications of moral emotions has been funded by NIDA, NICHD, NSF, and the John Templeton Foundation. Currently, her work focuses on moral emotions among incarcerated offenders. She draws on theory and research in psychology and criminology to develop novel interventions that leverage inmates' moral emotions and prosocial values.

JB: June, you are one of the relatively few empirical scholars in psychology who has studied and written on humility, especially from a twenty-first-century perspective, so I'd like to start with your understanding of it.

JPT: Well, humility isn't low self-esteem or the opposite of narcissism. It's really a construct unto itself rather than the opposite of something. It has to do with an accurate assessment of self, not overblowing or demeaning oneself. It's an attitude of "unselfing" where one is not the focus of attention but rather wants to learn and interact and focus on the outer world. The humble person is much less concerned about self-evaluation or others' evaluation of him or her. It's a willingness to be wrong and an interest in getting things right from others whom you readily admit might know more. The humble person doesn't engage in a lot of self-other comparison. They don't worry about how they rank with other people. There's a marked appreciation for other people, for their strengths and their weaknesses, which are most likely different from one's own. Because of that, a humble person doesn't think of others as better or worse; there's the belief that we all have a differing mix of talents and abilities.

JB: I'm recalling the phrase "optimal self-calibration," and I'm wondering if you wrote that or someone else.

JPT: No, that's not mine, but I love it.

JB: Do you think humility is catching on, especially given the descriptors you mentioned?

JPT: Well, I tend to think that humility is much more functional now given the enormous knowledge explosion than it was just a hundred years ago. When you think about lifelong learning, you didn't really need to have that in 1920, when the acquisition of knowledge was quite slow. But now we train people entirely differently. For example, I was trained in clinical psychology, and I can tell you that today we focus much more on empirically validated treatment. When I trained, I had one supervisor who was psychoanalytic, another who was humanistic, and another who was behavioral—and I had to make sense of all that with little guidance from data.

JB: So, you're emphasizing the knowledge acquisition part of this and the fact that a humble person realizes there's so little he or she knows and so much to learn.

JPT: Right, and that's a good thing.

JB: By the way, given that you and I both work on university campuses, do you think millennials are more or less narcissistic than their peers a generation ago? I've read some differing accounts among psychologists, and, of course, there's the ubiquitous selfie phenomenon.

JPT: That's a good empirical question, but I don't think that noting what may seem like certain narcissistic traits is the same as characterizing someone or some group as exhibiting a narcissistic disorder or pathology. In other words, I'm rather impressed with millennials in terms of their social involvement and their thinking about the world and humanity from a global perspective. The students in my classes are engaged and open minded. I'm pretty impressed with them.

JB: They give you hope for the future.

JPT: Yes, and I frankly don't see the narcissism among millennials that others claim to. However, I do worry that today, we have students taking college courses in their sophomore year in high school and others in seventh grade who are worried, along with their parents, about what will be on their résumés.

JB: Yes, we're living in an intensely hypercompetitive environment and having to deal with all the anxiety that comes with it. So I want to ask you whether you think that humility is more a product of nature than nurture? I believe you've said that humility is a pretty rare trait among human beings.

JPT: Oh, I didn't say that. If I did, I didn't mean it. I think like most personality traits, there's a distribution in a population as to how much or how little you have—and it's likely a normal distribution. In the Templeton group of humility researchers, one of the things we talk about is whether it makes sense to think of the trait humility across all domains—such as humility evenly expressed at work, in dealing with family, or in financial matters or social matters—or whether people vary in domains such that they have a lot of humility in some domains and less in others. Actually, there will be some answers to that fairly soon, as some Templeton researchers are generating data on that very question.

JB: What do you think people misunderstand about humility?

JPT: I think they think of it as low self-esteem or putting yourself down. We often think that people are humble when they say things like, "Oh, I'm such an awful baker. Everything I bake turns out badly." And they go on and on about how awful they are. Yet their conversation is entirely self-focused and very much comparison based with others and where they might rank. That isn't humility. The humble people I know listen and don't just talk; they observe equality in roles even though one person might be the mentor and the other the mentee. They're interested in exchanging ideas, not just imposing their ideas onto others. One of the things I'd love to look at is the interpersonal dimension that comes along with true humility. For example, I see some parents engaging their children in ways that show the parents' contempt for literally everything. Nearly everything the parent says to the child about the world is laced with skepticism, or they play devil's advocate, or everything is an argument. And so children have to respond assertively or confidently or else they're just blown away because that's what's being modeled.

JB: What do you think the prospects are for our health professionals becoming more humble in this twenty-first-century model?

JPT: I'd back up and say that when serious error occurs, we should analyze what happened and try to figure out ways to prevent future occurrences. To do this effectively, we need to be transparent, we need to not shame people, and we should admit how difficult it is to recognize a mistake and admit error. For the person who made the error, the question is, "How do I go forward from here and not make that mistake again and even share my experience with other people such as the junior people I'm teaching?" By the way, I suspect feelings of shame are inevitable, but the best strategy is to be looking to the future and figuring out the best ways to move forward. Of course, errors are inevitable, so we need to absorb that and then respond to them in a healthy way.

JB: So, I'd like to end by returning to what I think is one of the most interesting features of the humble personality—one that you already mentioned: that the humble person is somehow not self-preoccupied. In fact, I think you wrote in one of your articles that one of the methodological problems of doing research on humble people is that they don't care to talk about themselves.

JPT: Well, I suspect they don't know they're humble. They certainly don't know they are more humble than most people. They're not ranking themselves. But an important characteristic of humble people speaks to the difference between ambitious and competitive persons. Whereas the competitive person is always thinking about getting ahead of others, the ambitious person wants to get something done, and usually wants to share and learn with others. But I want to ask you a question.

JB: What's that?

JPT: You remarked in one of your emails about Mother Teresa and other folks who, on the one hand, demonstrate a lot of humility, but on the other, seem to enjoy the limelight. So, how do you understand that? Is there a good deal of narcissism here?

JB: So, I really like your distinction of competitiveness and ambition. I think Mother Teresa was a driven person, but for the sake of her values and the people she wanted to help. I don't think of her as a competitive kind of person, but then I don't know all that much about her. By the way, I also think of Oprah and Sully Sullenberger, the pilot who landed the plane on the Hudson, in this same regard. Again, I'm taken with your distinguishing ambition from competitiveness as quite revelatory of the way humble people—especially the very successful, publicly visible ones—think and react. Ultimately, though, all this might speak to the mystery of personality formation. You made the point that you can be humble in some domains but not humble in others. And I think the same goes for narcissism. Back when I trained in philosophy about 40 years ago, it was very common for scholars to say (and with a great deal of aplomb), "I am a Heideggerian" or "I am a Hegelian," which I always thought betrayed a great deal of narcissism. What they were doing was overidentifying with something, in this case a body of thought that they believed was powerful and magnificent.

JPT: Maybe data-driven people are different. At least if they are committed to where the data lead rather than because some philosopher argued for this or that, which they might resonate with. At least if you are committed to the data, assuming that the methodology is sound, then you might stand a better chance of getting at "the truth." Or if different points of view rest on different data, you can inquire into how the data were collected, what the key assumptions were, and all the things that inform one's methodology. Perhaps there's less room for defensiveness with that approach than with your example from the humanities.

JB: I became keenly aware of my narcissism when I reflected on how devastated I'd be when I got a manuscript rejected by a journal. It was such a blow to my ego, and it sometimes took me a week or two to recover. But I realized that there was something wrong with me to react like that. I knew it just wasn't healthy, but I think my ego was so brittle that a rejected manuscript felt like a rejected me.

JPT: And yet, one of the best and lasting ways to learn is by making mistakes and having them corrected. And I usually find that manuscript reviewers are or try to be objective and helpful, even though they are being critical, which is what we're asking them to do anyway.

JB: And you're right—that comports with my experience as well, but it's taken me too long to appreciate that. Now, it only takes me an hour to get over my homicidal rage when I get a rejection. Any last words?

JPT: Only that I'm delighted we're living in a more data-driven environment so that we can get an empirical handle on these difficult questions of personality formation. But as far as humility goes, I'm more hopeful about the future than I am discouraged. Really, that impression is one of the things that keeps me going.

JB: June, thank you so much.

JPT: You're welcome.

II   **Some Theoretical Musings
on Harm and Risk, Medical Error,
and Medical Malpractice Litigation
as an Ethical Exercise**

6 Some Theoretical Aspects of Vigilance and Risk Acceptability

What risks should we worry about? How do we know? What should we do about them? . . . Who decides what risks are of concern? Who is involved in assessing them? What is the role of science?

Dominic Golding and Seth Tuler[1(p2873)]

Chapter Overview. This chapter extends some of the theoretical points raised in chapter 2 on the nature of vigilance and risk reduction. A key question pervading the entire chapter is how much vigilance is owed by healthcare professionals to one another and to their patients. After briefly examining a response inspired by Harvard philosopher John Rawls's "veil of ignorance" heuristic, I argue that formula-based responses deriving from ethical theory will not provide helpful, practical answers. The reason is that the object of vigilance, namely, risk reduction, largely requires trial and error to know and manage. Our encounter with and learning about risk is continuously updated by experience and, moreover, is heavily contextualized: differing risk scenarios can require very different approaches. Theory, then, is too general to offer responses to risk reduction that will be practically helpful. The argument is supported by an example from the cancer literature involving morcellation surgery for uterine fibroid tumors.

Vigilance and Risk Reduction: How Much Can We Reasonably Demand?

Most risk conceptualizations present *risk* as a function of the probability and magnitude of an adverse event occurrence, that is, as the "measure of the likelihood and severity of harm resulting from a threat"; another characterization is "the quantitative measure of hazard consequence, usually expressed as conditional probabilities of experiencing harm."[1(p2873)] More recently, *velocity* has been added to the risk equation to account for how imminent the materialization of a risk is. Thus, the management of risk in healthcare involves (1) contemplating the probability, magnitude, and velocity of a harmful occurrence by (2) identifying the hazards that enable harm to occur; (3) developing control strategies to reduce the likelihood of hazard variables causing harm; (4) maintaining safe systems and practice behaviors, especially educative and corrective ones; and (5) maintaining and measuring outcomes so as to plan and implement quality-improvement and risk-reduction programs.[2]

Given these variables, the question of how much risk is acceptable in healthcare environments is a multifactorial one that involves ethical, sociological, psychological, and economic considerations. First, if eradicating or preventing the risk of some harm is within the reasonable control of system operators, then allowing that risk to persist would seem patently unethical. In Case 2.1 (acetylcysteine overdose), depositions of the treatment team revealed that they disagreed among themselves on what the X meant on the physician's (erroneous) medication order, although the institution's policy (as well as the national understanding) is that X means "times." (The confusion led to the 16-fold dosage error.) That kind of epistemic variation on such critical information as an X on a medication order is frankly outrageous and suggests a serious failure of the hospital's education programs. Similarly, when staff knowingly and intentionally violate rules, regulations, policies, and procedures whose function is to maintain patient safety, then violators should be held accountable and have extremely compelling reasons for such practice or protocol deviations (as discussed in chapter 4).

Once a practitioner or team has ramped up their safety sensibilities and practices to high levels of safety, however, they will find further risk reduction becomes increasingly difficult. They will now find themselves dealing with subtler or nonobvious variables that have been engineered into human cognition and behavior, as well as into the external environment toward which their attention is directed. They may experience confrontations with clinical and operational situations that are unprecedented, such that one doesn't know what risk variables are present, how they interact, and whether system operators will need additional resources (or just hope for dumb luck) to get through. And we all live in a world of wacky, unpredictable happenings for which no strategic knowledge exists and every, often improvised, response we create rests on a hope and a prayer. Risk reduction is extraordinarily contextualized: fall-prevention programs will use very different vigilance and risk-reduction strategies from those geared toward preventing nosocomial infections, while preventing sexual attacks in psychiatric settings will use different safety practices from those that focus on mitigating risks in an intensive care unit. Consequently, a one-size-fits-all answer to "How much vigilance we can reasonably demand?" or "How much risk reduction should we reasonably seek to achieve?" might be either unavailable or so vague or general as to be worthless.

Even so, philosophers have tried to answer the question of what vigilance and caution persons are owed; Anthony R. Reeves, for example, suggests we use John Rawls's "veil of ignorance" strategy to inform our intuitions about how safe our environments should be.[3] In his *A Theory of Justice*, the Harvard philosopher John Rawls used the metaphor of decision makers standing behind a "veil of ignorance" wherein they are charged with developing policies that distribute goods and benefits.[4] The decision makers must then live in that society without knowing (because they stand behind the veil deciding) what social positions or personal circumstances they will occupy once they find themselves at the receiving end of the distribution policies they create. Under such an arrangement, Rawls believed that rational, decent persons would reason according to their self-interests. But not knowing what socioeconomic position a person standing behind the veil will find him or herself in—rich man, poor man, beggar man, thief—he or she would likely favor a decent share of fundamental benefits for everyone and be inclined to protect individual liberties (or so Rawls thought).

Calling on our imaginations to consider the quality and extent of services we'd want in various situations of need is likely what often happens in a courtroom as jurors hear evidence and testimony on medical malpractice cases. They might well imagine themselves as patients in the defendant's clinic or hospital and ask whether they or any person would deem the care being described as acceptable, or acceptable enough. One hopes that they do not allow their knowledge of the plaintiff's outcome to affect their estimations of the defendants' innocence or guilt, since clinicians can do everything reasonably well and still witness a poor outcome. But if the opposing counsels have presented their evidence well and have chosen a reasonably intelligent jury, the outcome should be a just one. (I'll not entertain the ubiquitous physician complaint that only doctors should be on juries.)

Prospective healthcare consumers are perfectly reasonable to rely on the public promises made by professionals and institutions. We expect them to follow their own standards and guidelines; we are keenly aware of how dangerous healthcare provision is such that we insist on a high degree of training and excellence from its practitioners; and we inevitably use our knowledge acquired from managing risk in our own lives to assess the accountability of others. One hardly has to be an expert in risk management to take a very dim view of the hospital that did nothing about numerous and persisting complaints against a particular physician's conduct, or about multiple instances in which the same problem, such as unreliable technology, absent documentation, inadequate staffing, or similar situations, kept occurring but nothing was ever done to remediate the situation until disaster occurred.

But while this might give us a *negative* answer to how much vigilance patients are owed, that is, an attitude and set of practices that remediate behaviors or conditions that are *already recognized* as unreasonably harmful or ones that no reasonable person would want to risk, it doesn't respond substantively to how much vigilance should be built into the system, especially when those efforts begin witnessing "diminishing returns." Put otherwise and shifting the terminology from vigilance to its object, namely the recognition and reduction of hazard opportunities, organizations have no choice but to strike a balance between safety levels and productivity. Unfortunately, this tension is ineradicable because hiring additional staff, or investing in the best technology, or modifying a unit's architectural design might well enhance patient safety but substantially increase operational costs—some of which will be passed on to consumers. Consequently, an interesting exercise in moral values pertaining to patient safety might be to ask consumers, "How much safety are you willing to pay for?" rather than "What does ethics say should constitute a reasonably safe environment?" Nevertheless, in what follows I examine both questions.

Risk Reduction as a Choice with a Cost

Any industry, whether it be car manufacturing, energy, or food production, knows that risk/benefit trade-offs are inevitable. For example, the FDA permits up to 30 insect fragments in 100 grams of peanut butter, and 475 insect body parts per 50 grams of pepper.[5] Now, the numerator could be lowered with more pesticide use, but doing so not only would raise the price of the item but possibly increase health risks from pesticide exposure. Besides, consuming small amounts of insect parts, while seemingly disgusting, is not harmful.

Suppose, though, that a city's planners and leadership know that a particular intersection in town witnesses 10 percent more accidents on average than the town's other intersections. Further suppose that a safety analysis determined that an expenditure of $1 million would reduce the incidence of accidents to or below the city's average. Should the city raise taxes, resulting in, say, each city resident making a one-time payment of $10 to redesign the intersection? Would such an expenditure be "worth it"? Notice how much more information you'd need to make such a calculation—especially data on the severity of accidents occurring there, for example, are they fender benders or fatal crashes? Might better signage or better lighting reduce the accident rate somewhat but cost much less than $1 million? But by how much? And would that be "worth it"?

Economists love these kinds of thought experiments: for example, suppose there are 20 percent more accidents at the intersection rather than 10 percent, and it would cost $750,000 to fix the intersection; or that there was only a 5 percent increase in (very serious) accidents that would cost $3 million to remediate. Further suppose that the city's leadership has a long list of items that also require economic expenditures, like improving roads, bridges, or sewage systems. These are also risks that the reasonably vigilant person will want to consider. But life is replete with risks, and we simply lack adequate resources to remediate them all.

Another complicating factor is that a major determinant in an individual's willingness or unwillingness to pay for risk reduction will be his or her appetite for risk, which varies from person to person. People knowingly take remarkable risks—smoking, overeating, operating dangerous machines like motorcycles, and so on—but they might decry state-sponsored efforts that would diminish their risk taking as inimical with the individual liberties a liberal democracy promises. To be fair, though, such scenarios are disanalogous to those in healthcare, where patients are exposed to a hospital environment with its inherent risks not of their making, while a decision to ride a motorcycle or smoke is entirely one's own. Thus, we return to the originating question of this chapter, which is what professionals who are responsible for their service environments owe users by way of safety.

The argument that I pursue in the following pages is that this question cannot be settled according to philosophical or ethical theory. Rather, it can only be answered by trial-and-error experimentation, wherein system users implement practices and technologies that they have reason to believe are sufficiently safe and efficacious but that will need to be confirmed by experience, or trial and error. They will then use their values to determine which of those risks can be tolerated and which ones not. This means that an inherent problem regarding risk awareness in healthcare environments (or the level of vigilance responsibilities we can require of healthcare professionals) is the imperfection of human operators—especially in terms of constraints on their knowledge, judgment, and competence relative to the specific tasks they perform—and the enormous variation in values pertinent to risk aversion and tolerance. Those limitations are ineradicable from the human predicament and will continue until humans are replaced by technology whose functioning is vastly superior. The upshot of this observation is that philosophical or theoretical formulations of what would constitute an ideally acceptable risk threshold are compromised by real-world limitations, especially epistemological and economic ones, that render them impractical. I illustrate this argument with a sad but illuminating story.

The Imperfection of Risk Calculation and Risk Management

Consider the evolution (and apparent end) of morcellation technology in the treatment of uterine fibroid tumors and its challenge to "risk acceptability":

Case 6.1. Amy Reed, an anesthesiologist and intensive care physician, had been suffering from uterine fibroids and elected to have them removed via laparoscopy, a minimally invasive surgical procedure using small incisions through which the fibroid and uterine tissue are chopped up and vacuumed out.[6] Because laparoscopy is a closed rather than an open procedure, it does less damage to tissue, the surgery is faster and cheaper, the healing time is much more rapid than after an open procedure, and the risk of complications, such as pain and bleeding, surgical infections, and cosmetic disfigurement, is substantially reduced.

In removing Reed's tumors, her gynecologist used a *power morcellator*, which is a device consisting of a spinning blade that slices and dices the tissue into "morsels." In 2013, when Reed's operation occurred, physicians were using morcellators in 100,000 to 200,000 uterine fibroid surgeries per year.

An acknowledged risk of morcellation was that the sliced tissue could fly off the spinning blade and infiltrate adjacent or nearby anatomical areas. Consequently, if the fibrous tumor contained an aggressive cancer, which in a small number of cases it did, there was a risk that those cancer cells would take hold and create an *upstaging* (or increasing severity) of the original cancer. The risk of an aggressive cancer hiding in a uterine fibroid, however, was thought in 2013 to be extremely low, perhaps 1 in 10,000, such that the benefit-burden ratio seemed to very much favor morcellation.

A week after Reed's surgery, however, her surgeon contacted her with dreadful news. The pathology report came back positive for a *leiomyosarcoma*, which is an extremely aggressive cancer. In an open procedure, where the involved tissue would have been removed whole, a leiomyosarcoma patient's survival probability to 5 years would have been at least 50 percent. With the sarcoma morcellated, however, the 5-year survival odds dropped to 15 to 20 percent. Complicating the prognosis, it was reported that at the time of her surgery, Reed's leiomyosarcoma was staged at level IV, meaning that her 5-year survival rate was more like 14 percent. Thus, whether the use of morcellation reduced her survival odds or *made no difference to her survival* is a significant question in how much risk she was actually exposed to.[7] Reed succumbed to cancer on May 24, 2017.[8]

Almost immediately following her surgery, though, Reed's husband, Hooman Noorchashm, who is also a physician, commenced an intense study of morcellation in uterine fibroid surgery and began making disquieting findings about its risk. Other studies followed and cast morcellation in a much less favorable light than was originally thought, with findings like these:

- While the odds of a sarcoma in uterine fibroids is probably quite low among women without symptoms—perhaps approaching the 1-in-10,000 estimate Reed was initially told—an FDA study would later quote the odds at around 1 in 352, and with a leiomyosarcoma, 1 in 498 *among women whose fibroids cause severe symptoms as Reed's did.*[9]
- Noorchashm and Reed felt betrayed by one of her physicians, Michael Muto, who reportedly quoted the 1 in 10,000 risk of an aggressive cancer hiding in a fibroid. Muto had been an author on a study appearing about a year before Reed's surgery, where the researchers found unexpected sarcomas in 10 out of 1,091 tissue samples of women undergoing morcellation, prompting them to observe "an apparent associated increase in mortality much higher than appreciated currently."[10] Also, a South Korean study in 2011 showed that morcellation of leiomyosarcomas more than doubled the death rates compared with women having their tumors removed via laparotomy.[11]
- The FDA had never required any premarket testing of morcellators in women with fibroids, as the device had been grandfathered into use in the early 1990s because of its similarity with surgical devices already FDA approved.[6]
- When morcellators were used in other surgeries, physicians often attached a bag to the morcellator to catch the cut-up tissue. Yet, the FDA did not require the bag to be used, while Johnson and Johnson, the largest manufacturer of power morcellators (although not the maker of the one used on Reed) recommended using the bag when cancer was suspected. Johnson and Johnson did not manufacture such a bag, however.[6]

Noorchashm launched a virtual crusade against morcellation for uterine fibroid surgery, and in December 2013, the *Wall Street Journal* published a front-page article on Reed's surgery and its aftermath.[12] That article was followed by an editorial in the *Journal of the American Medical Association* warning about the risks of morcellation, followed by various hospitals announcing that they were limiting its use.[13] The FDA then followed with its own risk-benefit investigation of morcellation, and in April 2014, it issued an advisory opinion that discouraged the use of power morcellators in uterine fibroid surgery, quoting a 1 in 350 risk of sarcoma.[14] That claim, however, was opposed by representatives from the American College of Obstetricians and Gynecologists and the American Association of Gynecologic Laparoscopists, who argued that laparoscopic procedures remained safer than abdominal surgeries.[6] In July 2014, Johnson and Johnson nevertheless withdrew its morcellators from the market, and various insurers announced that they would not reimburse the costs of fibroid surgeries and hysterectomies where morcellators were used.[6] In November 2014 the FDA issued a black box warning on power morcellators, claiming them contraindicated for uterine fibroid surgery.[15]

In the meantime, Noorchashm and Reed filed lawsuits against Reed's hospital, various physicians, and the morcellator manufacturer Karl Storz. Defendants have either admitted no wrongdoing or have moved to dismiss the suits. Meanwhile, Johnson and Johnson has settled about 70 lawsuits from patients who alleged injury from the company's power morcellators and will likely settle more.[6]

Readers may feel that, given the above, the risk of harm from morcellation in uterine fibroid surgery seems unreasonably high. Indeed, many hospitals and clinicians have stopped using or offering morcellation to women with uterine fibroids. Yet, the debate about morcellator use, its statistical risk analyses, and a woman's right to choose the kinds of risks she deems acceptable remains ongoing.

Lisa Rosenbaum, a physician and correspondent for the *New England Journal of Medicine*, noted in the journal in 2016 that dismissing a woman's right to choose morcellation may be a violation of her autonomy and represents a capitulation to the "sensational anecdote gone viral" phenomenon rather than to a factual or data-driven argument.[16] Rosenbaum asked her readers to consider a young patient for whom a 6- to 8-week recovery from an open procedure for uterine fibroids would take a considerable economic and physical toll. If we respond that preventing her risk of death from cancer is well worth that cost, Rosenbaum might present other data that argue differently. She cites an article by Matthew Siedhoff and his colleagues, who published a decision tree analysis in a 2015 issue of the *American Journal of Obstetrics and Gynecology*, claiming that of 100,000 surgeries on women with presumptively benign fibroids, 98 would die from laparoscopy using morcellation, while 103 would die from an open procedure. More would die from morcellation than from an open approach, however, if a leiomyosarcoma were present (32 versus 12).[17]

A major variable in this benefit-burden calculation is the age of the patient. A younger woman rather than a peri- or postmenopausal woman probably has a much smaller chance of a sarcoma, such that Rosenbaum's hypothetical patient's opting for laparoscopy may not be unreasonable given the economic burdens and physical discomforts an open procedure would present. Rosenbaum argues that the risk-benefit trade-offs each procedure presents are genuinely problematic, and that ultimately a woman's autonomy should win out.

But an additional player in the doctor-patient relationship is also worried about risk: the healthcare institution. When I spoke with some gynecologists about risk and morcellation, one mentioned to me that her institution no longer allows the technology. This is an interesting twist in the saga of risk assumption: Are healthcare institutions banning the use of morcellation with a paternalistic eye to diminishing an excessive or unallowable level of risk to female patients, or do these hospitals primarily want to reduce their liability and so deny the morcellation treatment option to women undergoing fibroid surgery? And how much information exists that would enable a hospital or clinic to feel confident about its decision, assuming that the decision is ethically motivated and not simply a hyper, hospital-centered, risk-averse response?

What Does This Case Teach about Risk Acceptability?

Assuming that I have related Dr. Reed's case in a factually accurate way, it appears to present a host of factors that traverse the landscape of risk knowledge and choice, beginning with certain decisions that appeared reasonable but that then vectored to risk knowledge that was flawed and inaccurate (and so was not "knowledge" at all); to marked differences among experts on risk taking and on risk perception; to securing what might have been more accurate risk information but whose content was not widely known and hence not incorporated into the standard of care; to power brokers who had to weigh economic variables into the mix of deciding which risks are acceptable and which ones not; to reformulations of risk knowledge and awareness; and finally to the tension between a patient's autonomy in the face of risk versus an institutional authority's power to ignore that freedom and impose its own vision of "safety."

Consider that in terms of what was widely known and practiced when Reed first appeared for her surgery, a laparoscopic approach done with a power morcellator seemed reasonable. It was the treatment of choice because the risk of an aggressive cancer hiding in a uterine fibroid was thought extremely low. Tragically, Reed was the victim of cruelly bad luck in that her tumor hid an aggressive cancer, but the use of the morcellator possibly made no difference in her ultimate outcome since her cancer was already advanced.

Emerging knowledge from the FDA, however, would revise all those early risk calculations, as new research altered the odds of a sarcoma from 1 in 10,000 to 1 in 350 to 500 among women with symptoms like Reed's. Had that knowledge been widely available when Reed first appeared for surgery, *it is impossible to imagine that her surgery would have proceeded laparoscopically.*

We also had the problematic appearance of some research, appearing a year before Reed's surgery, suggesting that the risk of an aggressive cancer hiding in a fibroid was much higher than originally thought. But that knowledge was not communicated to Reed by one of the physicians who treated her, even though that very person was reportedly aware of that data, as he was one of the researchers who discovered it. Did he believe his findings were uncertain or tentative—at least to the point of not challenging the extant standard of care that favored morcellation?

If we know one thing about the standard of care, however, it is that it can be robustly subject to frequent revision. Vinay Prasad and his colleagues, for example, reported that of 363 journal articles they reviewed over a 10-year period (2001-2010) that tested a standard of care, 146 standards have been reversed.[18] Consequently, an initial and persuasive calculation of safety and efficacy is hardly assured.

Returning, then, to our initial question of how much vigilance or risk reduction patients and families are owed, if a case like Amy Reed's is at all generalizable to how knowledge about vigilance, hazard awareness, and risk reduction in healthcare actually develops, then theoretical or philosophical arguments drawing on abstract formulations of harm or justice will not deliver answers that are useful or practical. To see this, we can return to Rawls's veil of ignorance and ask those standing behind the veil how much risk healthcare consumers should assume. If, however, our very comprehension of the nature and gravity of those risks under consideration is uncertain or unreliable, as it was in Amy Reed's case, then the decision makers can only make decisions that strike them as the best that can be made at that moment. Not only will they have an incomplete knowledge of the practical or real-life context in which those risks occur, but their informants will be without an adequate knowledge base that frames how harm or justice should figure in their determinations. To even put the question on "the degree of vigilance" that is owed up for philosophical speculation or debate would therefore be unfair because we lack the specific risk data that would inform what system operators should be vigilant about or toward. The best we can do, then, is what humans have been doing for tens of thousands of years: experiment with what we suspect might be adaptive interactions with our environments, carefully note the results, pass on our accumulated wisdom to others, and continue that knowledge confirmation, but proceed in all this with a spirit of epistemic fallibility.

Risk knowledge, especially recently evolved risk knowledge, can be remarkably wrong, and in either direction: too unappreciative and ignorant of serious risk lurking in the performance environment, or overly cautious where one needn't be. Decades of experience with risk, especially as it applies to patient safety, direct more worry to the former than to the latter. Humans, especially working in complex performance environments, are often less wary of risk than they should be, perhaps because an unnecessarily risk-averse attitude will become self-evident and aware of its needless excesses and wearisome energy expenditures and give way, through experience, to more efficient but just as safe attitudes and practices. In all this, however, theory will be of little use in shaping the navigation of that risk environment. What learners will instead depend on is knowledge accumulated through trial and error, experienced teachers, and a humble willingness to regard their risk knowledge as tentative.

The Risk Management Department

The heart of the risk conscience in a hospital is the risk management or patient safety department, whose job it is to monitor and consider mitigation of *all* risks.[2] These risks include not just patient safety risks, but organizational risks (e.g., making strategic decisions for surviving in the marketplace), financial (e.g., keeping a lid on medical malpractice premium costs), workforce risks (e.g., employee selection, on-the-job injury, retention, turnover, absenteeism), regulatory issues (e.g., monitoring fraud and abuse, accreditation, compliance with Medicare and Medicaid services, safe medication practices), technology (e.g., electronic health records), and hazard (e.g., facility management, parking, windstorm damage, floods, etc.).[19] Risk management is the "vigilance center" of the organization's sensitivity to risk and assumes the roles of "prevention, reduction, and control of loss to the health organization."[19(p120)]

Although risk managers are frequently trained as health professionals, especially nurses, their role is largely not a clinical one but an information-gathering, analytical, policy-making, and educational one. Risk management receives reports from various institutional committees charged with patient safety, such as quality assurance and infection control, survey reports like the Joint Commission's, and claims data from the organization's insurers. Of course, risk management receives incident reports of things gone wrong and failures to follow standards of care, and risk managers track *sentinel events*—which are usually understood as "never events" and are reportable to accrediting agencies like the Joint Commission and patient safety organizations like the Institute for Safe Medication Practices.[20] Most importantly, risk management performs failure mode and effect analysis, which seeks to identify harm threats and eliminate them before adversity occurs.[19]

The data collection and analysis functions that risk management performs recalls the wisdom of James Reason's comment in the previous chapter on the importance of a patient safety reporting culture, because if risks are not identified and known, they cannot be addressed and controlled: "Neither commitment nor competence will suffice unless the organization is adequately cognizant of the dangers that threaten its activities. Cognisant organizations understand the true nature of the struggle for enhanced resilience. For them, a lengthy period without adverse events does not signal 'safe enough'. They see it correctly as a period of heightened danger and so review and strengthen their defences accordingly. In short, cognizant organisations maintain a state of intelligent wariness even in the absence of bad outcomes. This is the very essence of a safe culture."[21(p274)]

Although risk management is keen to eliminate risks of high likelihood and high impact, other variables that affect risk-management efforts include the amount of resources needed to control risk, the challenges and benefits of the effort, how operationally complex a risk-reduction program might be, and what would constitute a reasonable time line for implementation.[1,19]

Consequently, *risk acceptability*, or tolerance, is essentially an ethical challenge because, at least theoretically, no preventable clinical risk is acceptable. Yet, mitigating all risks is impossible, so the organization must make
various value-laden decisions about where to commit its safety resources.
Furthermore, because actual risk calculations are heavily detailed and contextualized, the application of ethical principles in the pursuit of ethical
wisdom may be of limited value because their abstractness does not reach
the fine-grained particularity that such on-the-ground decisions require.

Conclusion

This chapter continues the argument that patient safety ethics requires a
different approach from the familiar one of traditional bioethics. In patient
safety, conceptions of rights, harms, benefits, and justice seem challenged in
unfamiliar ways, yet intellectual reflection and analysis should find a solution that moral logic endorses. While the context of patient safety inevitably
uses the language of ethical principles, however, the dynamic interface of
performance competence, uncertainty, and highly variable work contexts
are inimical with armchair speculations that seek to resolve their quanda-
ries. Aristotle would say that the knowledge involved in patient safety is in-
eluctably phronetic, which, as Albert R. Jonsen and Stephen Toulmin put it,

> concerned concrete situations the nature and complexity of which were un-
> known beforehand: it dealt with them not by merely reapplying predetermined
> generic techniques but by recognizing what combinations of actions are appro-
> priate to complex or ambiguous situations . . . [C]linical physicians have no spe-
> cific predefined tasks because their responsibility is to deal perceptively and in
> a timely way with whatever medical needs any particular patient may have, in
> response to all eventualities, as and when they may occur. This . . . kind of "prac-
> tical" knowledge, Aristotle says, is exemplified in the capacity to deal with the
> moral demands of life in perceptive and timely ways, as and when they arise. This
> puts ethics into the realm of phronesis, "prudence," or "practical wisdom."[22(p65)]

As such, the ethical contours of patient safety will perforce require practical
know-how guided by medicine's Hippocratic sensibility of doing no unnecessary harm. What propels our inquiries into the arena of prudential wisdom is that neither practical know-how nor a sensibility committed to not
harming can proceed without an intelligence largely trained by experiential
knowledge, one that knows what to do and why to do it in the specific circumstance that is presented. Although grounded in an ethic of patient cen-

teredness, as is all healthcare, patient safety and its associated obligations occur through the manipulation of the patient's surroundings, especially as they incline toward hazards and risks. Yet the nature of the latter is not generic but particular through and through, and only by repeated and intense encounters with those particulars can safety wisdom and its accompanying ethical formation occur.

7   Fifty Shades of Error

We're trained from our earliest days in school that health professionals don't make mistakes, and if you do, you don't talk about it.

Mary Ann Ayd, quoting Beryl Rosenstein[1(p25)]

One has to wonder why we doctors feel our entire sense of self at risk when we admit error. Perhaps the culture of perfection in medicine fosters a strictly binary analysis: You're either an excellent doctor or a failure. In most other aspects of life, we seem to be able to accept the notion of "good enough."
But there is no room for the good-enough doctor.

Danielle Ofri[2]

Chapter Overview: This chapter provides a wide-ranging discussion of medical error. It begins with a definition of error and differentiates error from harm. I then proceed to discuss various error-related topics, including debates over the incidence of fatal medical error in the United States, the dense contextuality of a serious medical error, and the bewildering array of error types. A perennial topic in error studies is disclosing the error to involved parties. I offer arguments for why error should be disclosed, but also why that disclosure can be psychologically difficult and complicated by numerous clinical details (and, oftentimes, disagreements). I conclude with a discussion of incident reporting, the need to involve patients and families in risk-reduction efforts, and an interview with Fran Charney, the current (2018) director of risk management for the American Society for Healthcare Risk Management.

Defining Error

A popular definition of error relies on intention, as in "error may be defined as an unintended act . . . or one that does not achieve its intended outcome."[3(p1851)] But as I and others have argued, this is a poor definition, because reality can always surprise us with situations that defy our intentions and their anticipated outcomes but not implicate error. The surgeon who accidentally nicks an adjacent anatomical structure obviously didn't plan or intend for that to happen, but if the patient's anatomy is very complex or the surgical site is marred by scarring or adhesions from previous surgeries, the nick might be all but unavoidable and hence not an error. A physician is certainly not intending to cause an anaphylactic shock when he orders an antibiotic. But with no good reason to have anticipated such a reaction from the patient, the doctor cannot be said to have erred by providing the medication. Rather, we would call these adversities "complications."

A better although not perfect definition is to characterize error as an unacceptable, unallowable, or palpably suspect departure from what one ordinarily or reasonably should do or should have done. In other words, error is an unjustifiable departure from the standard of care.[4] On that basis, error sounds very much like what the law calls "negligence" and recalls a previous observation: the standard of care not only expresses what patients are owed, but also differentiates error from non-error.

In my experience, health professionals bristle at the suggestion that error equates to negligence, probably because negligence sounds perverse and litigious, while error sounds more human and perhaps forgivable. But it would be better, especially in healthcare, to admit that when one errs, even in making an "honest mistake" (which I suppose implies that the mistake was unintentional or that it could have been made by anyone), one has almost certainly violated the standard of care, that is, done something an ordinary, reasonable professional would not have done in a similar situation. As one malpractice lawyer put it, "The health care provider is negligent if and only if he has acted unreasonably, i.e., done something no reasonable health care provider would have done under the circumstances. Whether an act (or failure to act) by a health care professional is reasonable can only be analyzed under the specific circumstances of the case."[5]

Errors in medicine, therefore, need not cause any harm except if they are being litigated, where the burden of proof is on the plaintiff to prove *harm-causing* error.[5] I err when I misstate a bioethical argument or a legal case in class, even though my error probably harms no one. Nurse Williams errs when she administers the wrong medication to patient Diaz, who suffers no harm from it. Pathologist Henderson errs when he confuses specimens from two patients, although, luckily, no harm occurs to either one. None of these cognitive or psychomotor failures should have happened, but they do because humans are prone to memory failure, inattention, haste, inexperience, poor communication, faulty technique, flawed knowledge, cognitive bias, applying the wrong conceptual or behavioral schema, exercising poor judgment, and the list goes on and on.[6]

The unsettling ethical point in all this is that authentic errors are breaches of a clinician's obligation to reasonably ensure patient safety. This may be hard to accept because it sounds impossibly stern, but the logic is inexorable: If health professionals have a prima facie obligation to care for patients according to whatever professional standards are in place, then they most likely err if they fail to do so. Alternatively, health professionals are on entirely defensible grounds if they can show that they were reasonably compliant with rules and standards despite a disappointing outcome. Furthermore, if the professional does deviate from the standard but can give a very persuasive reason for doing so, then more likely than not, the standard wasn't contextually applicable to begin with. In any event, I'm proposing that whichever standards of care contextually and reasonably apply should serve as ethically objective reference points that differentiate error from non-error, regardless of whether harm occurred.

In chapter 3, I surveyed the idea of mindfulness as an ethical construct in patient safety, so it's important to ask whether professionals practicing mindfulness strategies can still err. They can, of course, because even scrupulous attention to the possibility of error won't guarantee its nonoccurrence. How often are we superbly confident of our judgment or belief and cannot believe it to be erroneous even though it was? Perhaps we scrutinized and checked that table of calculations or spreadsheet of data multiple times for errors but later learn we made them anyway.

At best, mindfulness will enable us to reduce the frequency and severity of harm-causing errors but not entirely eliminate them. In this chapter, however, I do envision not the mindful healthcare provider but the one who is sailing through his or her day largely engaged in System 1 thinking. Fortunately, System 1 will usually serve this person and his or her patients well enough. Yet, it seems that most errors occur amid System 1 cognition and that most mindfulness strategies represent System 2 thinking. In the pages that follow, I examine the occurrence of error not only as the thoroughly human phenomenon it is but according to the multiple ways in which it occurs in healthcare cultures. I begin with some observations on the language and contexts of error, as well as their all-too-numerous manifestations. Despite the dozens of very good papers on error disclosure, I cannot resist including a few of my own thoughts on it, given the challenges that disclosure continues to pose to health professionals. Presumably, incident reporting constitutes an indispensable database for learning about the circumstances of error, yet it too continues to present a compliance challenge for health professionals. Taken together, this brace of topics illustrates why not only error commission but its aftermath remain a source of conflict and challenge for realizing the ethical dimensions of patient safety goals.

Error Admission as Self-Incrimination

Semantic considerations of the meaning of error are not merely academic niceties but important elements in a health provider's knowledge base when an adverse event requires disclosure to a patient or his or her family. Calling X an error amounts to calling a foul on oneself. It is essentially to say, "I/we screwed this up. This should not have happened because it was reasonably preventable, but we allowed it to happen. It was our fault, and we are very sorry."[7]

The word "fault" is why twentieth-century hospital attorneys and the hospital's defense attorneys would cringe if a clinician uttered the word "error" to a patient, because such an admission was frequently understood as tantamount to admitting guilt and imperiling the professional's and institution's liability.[8] Indeed, twentieth-century historical anecdotes abound of health professionals being explicitly told by someone from "legal" never to say the words "error" or "mistake" and never to apologize to a patient or family for what happened. Given that many of those health professionals wouldn't want to conduct an error disclosure conversation in the first place, such recommendations for error concealment from the institution's legal authorities must have been very welcome. It is small wonder that the twentieth century wasn't notable for significant advances in patient safety given the career-suicide connotations of error disclosure among health professionals. Nevertheless, in an ideally just society, the only errors that would come to the attention of malpractice courts would be the harm-causing ones, because plaintiffs must be proximately harmed by error (or negligence) for their malpractice actions to proceed.[9(p9)]

This is illustrated by Case 1.1, in which the patient received a drug to which she had a documented allergy and then died 48 hours later. Within 90 minutes after taking the drug, she developed typical drug reaction symptoms—shortness of breath, hives, itching—and 24 hours later appeared to be developing Stevens-Johnson syndrome, from which she died the following day. Although an allergy to sulfa is one of the leading causes of Stevens-Johnson, there's usually a latency period of at least 4 days.[10,11] Her nearly immediate Stevens-Johnson-like reaction to the drug was therefore quite unusual, although she had been taking other drugs during her hospitalization that could have also caused the syndrome. Alternatively, many patients in acute care hospitals are extremely ill such that it may be next to impossible to say with any degree of certainty whether a patient's demise was caused by an error or by the patient's underlying pathology. Juries simply use their best judgment in determining causality and, of course, are often influenced by extra-evidential factors, such as their like or dislike of the defendants, plaintiffs, experts, or the attorneys. In any event, I shall go to my grave wondering about whether the sulfa drug caused this patient's demise. Fortunately for the plaintiffs, the case settled, perhaps suggesting that the defendants did not wish to attempt to disprove the plaintiff's sulfa-causation argument in court.

Are Medical Errors the Third Leading Cause of Death in the United States?

In the May 2016 issue of *BMJ*, Martin Makary and Michael Daniel argued that, based on several very recent studies, medical error appears to be the third leading cause of death in the United States, just after cardiac disease and cancer.[12] While the most commonly cited statistic on fatal medical errors is the 1999 IOM report of 44,000 to 98,000 yearly deaths, Makary and Daniel noted that this number and, indeed, all estimations since were based on extrapolations from acute hospital statistics. Fatal errors occurring at primary care clinics, nursing homes, rehabilitation hospitals, and same-day surgery centers weren't included, leading epidemiologists to estimate that a more accurate count of error-related deaths might be somewhere between 210,000 to 400,000 a year.[13]

Although others have disputed Makary and Daniel's estimates, any error-related death in theory should be preventable, along with the hundreds of thousands of nonfatal but serious error-related harms that also occur.[14] Error remediation begins with an organizational commitment to attend to such occurrences and their enabling factors, advice that wasn't embraced during most of the twentieth century, presumably because error-related harms and deaths were embarrassing and upsetting, and fears over liability drove such conversations underground. As such, health professionals unwittingly deprived themselves of the opportunity to learn from errors— their circumstances, causal and harming factors, trajectories, and outcomes. Today, learning from error occurrence is an ethical imperative. We need especially to know what it was like to be the person primarily involved in the error, especially regarding the cognitive demands of the task and its environmental constraints or conditions. What variables allowed the error to occur and then go undetected? What system factors would likely have detected the error and intercepted it so that its harm potential could have been defused? In short, what can a root cause (or causes) analysis tell us about safety improvement?

Granularity: Error-Related Harms Are Extremely Contextual

Recently, various insurers, along with the Centers for Medical Services, were threatening institutions that allowed sentinel events to occur—such as skin breakdowns, wrong-side surgeries, retained instruments following surgery, patient falls, and so forth—with refusing to reimburse treatment costs associated with the event.[15] Sentinel event occurrences invariably cast a suspicious eye toward the treating clinicians, whose actions or inactions may have enabled these presumably preventable events. The pain of revenue loss is hoped to incentivize greater efforts to advance patient safety, along with, of course, the threat of medical malpractice suits for harm caused by negligence.

The scholarly literature suggests, however, that simply telling people to "be more careful" or to "pay more attention" is ineffective, especially among adult professionals who already are reasonably dependable and skilled.[16] Reducing errors among this population will likely require environmental change, such as installing less complex and more user-friendly technology and removing ecological variables that make us vulnerable to error commission, like hunger, stress, dim lighting, inadequate training, distractions, unreasonable productivity quotas, better communication with staff and patients, and so on.

One of the most challenging features of reducing error-related harms is their degree of particularity, or contextualization. For example, the Institute for Safe Medication Practices lists hundreds of soundalike drugs (see "List of Confused Drug Names," https://www.ismp.org/recommendations /confused-drug-names-list) that unfortunately make for excellent error opportunities. But being on guard not to confuse Adderall with Inderal is no guarantee that one won't confuse primidone with prednisone. And even if a hospital completes a training effort such that nurses scrupulously practice the five Rs of medication delivery—right patient, right medication, right dose, right route, right time—that training measure will not reduce the hospital's fall rate or the number of missed infections in the emergency room.

And this situation is a primary reason that the attempt to reduce error-related harms is so frustrating despite the patient safety movement launch in 1999. Error-related harms are highly contextualized because of the unique cluster of variables that populates and defines a given clinical situation. Improvements in one context, like reducing radiology misinterpretations, cannot be expected to spill over into another error context, like timely medication delivery. But perhaps even more upsetting is how the variables within a given context or clinical situation may change from day to day and disorient treating professionals. Richard Cook has succinctly observed, "[I]nnovation introduces new forms of failure," such that everyone should be hyperwary of the first time a novel technology is used.[17] James Reason, on the other hand, wants to call attention to how that novelty plays out within a work environment already beset by suboptimal organizational and cognitive processes, involving "fatigue, technical problems, high work load, poor communication, conflicting goals, inexperience, low morale, teamwork deficiencies, etc."[18(p59)]

The relentless introduction of novelty virtually assures the commission of error-related harms: new drugs and devices, interventions, technologies, personnel, policies and regulations, documentation, and information systems all overlap in practice to meet production quotas without, one hopes, compromising safety. To the extent that the healthcare environment witnesses relentless, qualitative change requiring new learning among system operators, errors are simply inevitable. As James Reason memorably noted, "Safety is a guerrilla war that you will probably lose . . . [T]he only attainable safety goal is not zero accidents, but to strive to reach the zone of maximum practicable resistance and then remain there for as long as possible."[19(pp288,285)]

Thus, while I extol the virtues of mindfulness in a previous chapter, these environmental variables, especially associated with innovation, illustrate its limits. Although the more mindful we are, the better, error opportunities can arise in our performance and exploit our imperfect cognitive equipment in simply too many ways. Thus, the ongoing need to supplement cognitive practices like vigilance and mindfulness with technological, leadership, and relational tools and approaches (like involving patients and their families in the clinical reasoning process) to reduce the frequency and magnitude of error.

The Bewildering Array of Errors

There may be 50 shades of gray, but there are thousands of ways to commit medical error:

- *At least five generic kinds of medication errors.* The as-ordered medicine delivered to the wrong patient; the wrong medicine delivered to the right patient; the wrong route—such as an intramuscular injection being given rather than an intravenous injection; wrong dosage; wrong time at administration.[20] Notice that each of these error types can be caused by a multitude of related error opportunities—for example, the wrong patient received the medicine because she had a soundalike name, or the nurse forgot to check her armband or to look at the drug label.

- *At least three different kinds of diagnostic errors.* The categorical, unjustified miss when the patient is told everything is fine, but, in fact, he or she has a serious ailment that should have been detected; false positives or false negatives, when patients with disease X are told that they have disease Y, or that they definitely don't have disease X when they do; and the delay, when a particular test should have been done, say, in January but isn't performed until November, allowing the patient's conditions to seriously worsen.[21]

- *Interpretation errors.* The examples are legion. In Jerome Groopman's book *How Doctors Think*, he tells a story about the noted radiologist Dennis Orwig.[22] The story goes that a colleague enters Orwig's office and shows him a knee scan. Orwig glances at it and declares it a "torn ACL"—anterior cruciate ligament, one of the most common of serious knee injuries. The physician points to the doctor's name who originally interpreted the scan. It's Orwig's, and he had misread it as a normal anterior cruciate ligament. Groopman reports Orwig saying, "I was mystified . . . It's incredible that at one time I could look at a film and only later see what I had missed."[22(p186)] Perhaps this isn't even an "interpretation" error but a perceptual miss. Yet, we commit these errors all the time, whether it's failing to notice the gorilla in front of the elevators (see "Missing the 200-Pound Gorilla in the Room," http://big think.com/videos/missing-the-200-pound-gorilla-in-the-room) or holding the refrigerator door open in search of the mayonnaise jar, which we're staring at but don't notice. The stakes are considerably higher in radiology, though, where, Groopman reports, "Even the best radiologists will inaccurately read a mammogram in 2 to 3 percent of the cases, while some studies show that other doctors incorrectly read the images in 20 percent or more."[22(pp187-88)]

- *Vigilance errors.* These are largely inattention or not-knowing-where-to-look errors. One of the most publicized involved the death of 18-month-old Josie King. This story is one of the "classic" tragedies in the medical error literature, in which Josie's mother, Sorrel King, noticed that her hospitalized daughter seemed severely dehydrated. Despite the mother's pleas to the nursing staff, she was ignored and told that her daughter's vital signs were fine. A nurse then injected Josie with a syringe of methadone, and Josie's heart stopped. Two days later, she was taken off life support and died. Sorrel King recalled, "Our lives were changed forever . . . Josie's death was not the fault of one doctor, or one nurse . . . It was the result of a complete lack of communication between the different teams. It was the result of doctors and nurses not listening to a concerned parent. It was the result of a combination of many errors, all of which were avoidable."[23]

- *Errors committed in haste.* We all recognize how our performance deteriorates when we accelerate beyond our comfort zones. In healthcare, a particularly worrisome example occurs in busy, high-activity, high-production environments in which health professionals are always behind and working feverishly to catch up. Disastrous diagnostic errors have been noted to occur from the confluence of two kinds of bias that are especially related to haste: the availability bias and the confirmation bias. Dr. Walters sees a patient with a particular symptom cluster that immediately starts him thinking, "This person has Q." Walters orders tests that appear to confirm Q, but he forgets that the tests also suggest diagnosis P, which his pressured or anxious thinking ignores. Because Q is usually what such patients have, he feels confident that the patient has Q. Also, he has dozens more patients he needs to see that day, and ordering and interpreting more tests is time consuming. Months go by, and the patient does not improve because he indeed has P, not Q. The more certain Walters is about Q, the more he resists considering alternative diagnoses or ordering more tests. Although this is an infrequent occurrence, if it occurs in only 1 to 5 percent of the patients Dr. Walters sees, at the end of the year, that number will be considerable.

- *Cognitive traps and pitfalls.* Consider this puzzle: "A baseball bat and a baseball together cost $1.10. The bat costs $1 more than the ball. How much does each item cost?"[24(p44)] The question, which a sixth-grader should get right, was circulated among undergraduates at Ivy League universities and at public universities. About 50 percent of the Ivy League students got it wrong, while more than 50 percent of the public university students got it wrong. The answer is that the bat costs $1.05, and the ball costs $0.05. If you said that the bat costs $1.00 and the ball costs $0.10, then the bat would cost $0.90 more than the ball. But you were told the bat costs $1.00 more. (Yes, I got it wrong as well.) If very simple problems like these trick us into error, what happens when we find ourselves in cognitively complex situations like emergency rooms, where the stakes are high and our cognition needs all the help it can get? If committing error in this or that situation is terribly easy, then the patient safety challenge is to make error commission *harder*, which may require considerable ingenuity and expense if the remedy requires architectural or workflow alterations.

- *Knowledge errors.* These errors are scary and very common. We want to think that clinical acumen is evenly distributed among our nation's physicians, but it isn't. Dr. Walters may be adept at diagnosing heart disease but not cancer. He might not know what tests to order when a patient presents with a certain cluster of symptoms, or he may order the correct tests but then not know what treatment plan he should launch after receiving the test results. Worse, he rarely gets feedback on his diagnostic mistakes, which lures him into thinking his diagnostic skills are superlative.

- *Assumption errors.* In Chassin and Becher's classic paper "The Wrong Patient," they describe a patient mix-up in which "Joan Morris" has a procedure—an electrophysiologic study with possible implantable cardiac defibrillator and pacemaker—that is actually scheduled for "Jane Morrison."[25] The root cause analysis identifies 17 separate errors, most of which involve communication failures. Lurking behind many of these communication failures, however, are what might be called "errors of assumption," such as the nurse who transports the patient from the floor to the operating room and notices the absence of an informed consent for the procedure but assumes the study is arranged; and a resident physician who is taking care of the patient and is similarly surprised that she has been taken to surgery for an electrophysiologic study. He simply assumes the test was ordered without the attending telling him. The nurse who receives the patient for the procedure also notices the absence of an informed consent for the procedure, and she pages the electrophysiology fellow who is participating in the procedure to check. The fellow is "surprised" at the lack of pertinent information regarding this patient and her need for the procedure—which is hardly surprising because she's the wrong patient—but he assumes everything is in order and gets the patient to sign the consent form. Throughout all this, the patient is telling the staff that no one mentioned to her a need for a cardiac examination but the staff ignores her.

Error Disclosure

Anecdotal evidence suggests that frank, truthful, transparent, and empathic disclosure of error was unusual in the twentieth century. Some recent surveys of patients or families who suffered adverse events suggest that incomplete, obfuscatory, or all too brief "disclosures" remain common if not the norm. A 2014 paper by Heather Lyu and her colleagues at Johns Hopkins surveying 236 patients who reported experiencing an iatrogenic harm and who filed a complaint with an oversight agency found that "only 9.3% of medical facilities and 7.6% of clinicians voluntarily disclosed the harm to patients and their families. Furthermore, only 11.4% of patients or their families received an apology from the facility or the provider . . . These low rates of disclosure and apology demonstrate the hesitation of health care workers to fully open the doors of communication with patients. A common explanation for the reluctance to disclose is that clinicians recognize the importance of disclosure but lack the moral courage to participate in an open discussion."[26(p200)]

Note, however, that the respondents in this study represented a self-selected group who reported having experienced what they perceived to be preventable harm, with 20 percent of them proceeding to sue. Consequently, the paper does not reflect the experience of other patients who may have been harmed from error but who chose not to file a report, possibly because they were satisfied with the way the institution handled their experience. We are left, then, with three possibilities for error discourse: (1) that an error is disclosed in an ideally empathic, comprehensive, and truthful fashion; (2) that it is disclosed halfway, with the professional withholding some information, such as omitting the words "error" or "mistake," and letting the family speculate or ask questions; or (3) that the error is not disclosed, suggested, or implied in any way.

Whichever of these occur, it seems safe to say that nothing puts an institution's public "patient-centered" or "transparency" declarations to the test like the disclosure of medical error. Reluctance over disclosing a serious, harm-causing error is a classic example of self-interest colliding with doing what is morally right. The literature reports that health professionals' reactions to error runs the psychological gamut: intense anguish that can end in the professional's leaving his or her career or, in very rare cases, committing suicide; a dull sadness and guilt that some clinicians bear throughout their careers; a not-all-that-painful learning experience that morphs over time into a memorable lesson in humility; or an experience that is rapidly dismissed and largely forgotten.[27]

Arguments for Disclosing Error

I have wondered about the best argument for disclosing error. Many health professionals might dismiss the most commonly offered one by the American Medical Association's Council on Ethical and Judicial Affairs, namely that patients have a right to know what happened so that they can subsequently make informed judgments about their care. The AMA's argument is that if the patient suffered error-related harm, he or she has a right to such information regardless of its impact on the health professional.[28(p8.12)] Although that might sound compelling, the professional can easily convince him or herself that delivering such information will psychologically harm the patient or the family. Also, professionals may point to the "cooperation prohibition" clause of their medical malpractice policy as forbidding disclosure. Such clauses state that if the policyholder admits liability for an event normally covered by the policy, the insurer may refuse to cover it.[29] The insurer's rationale is that by admitting liability—as might happen in the disclosure of error—the insured is depriving the insurer of an opportunity to defend the case and thus conserve the insurer's resources. Thus, insured health professionals sometimes argue that disclosure of error is simply too great a risk, because not only might it invite a lawsuit, it also might result in the insurer's refusing coverage for a legal defense and any settlement or jury award that results from litigation. According to this argument, the price of disclosure for the insured health professional is simply too great.[29]

A compelling ethical argument to counter this is that often today's patients and family members will suspect negligence when the reasonable anticipation of a positive outcome is greatly but mysteriously disappointed. Case 1.5 was such a situation: An otherwise healthy woman went in for a routine gall bladder operation, and things went terribly wrong. She experienced an anoxic episode during the operation as a result of an anesthesi-ologic error that went unrecognized by the surgical team and that plunged her into a vegetative state. Her well-educated adult children were never in-formed of the errors that caused her demise—she would be disconnected from artificial ventilation nine days later and expire two days afterward—yet they testified in their depositions that they felt the surgeon and anesthe-siologist were withholding vital information. In the surgeon's deposition, he admitted he could see their suffering and grief, especially stemming from their ignorance of what happened, but he believed that it was the anesthe-siologist's mistake and that the anesthesiologist should disclose. The family remained devastated because they were without a narrative that could bring some closure to their tragedy. When they finally learned of the anesthesi-ologic error, their anguish and rage erupted. One hears this story often: The patient and/or family are plunged into unrelenting misery over what happened because the institution cannot marshal its courage and resources to effect an ethical disclosure of error. While the institution may well have a host of explanations for that failure—such as the physician claiming that error did not occur; no one being willing to disclose an error that clearly did occur; the communication being very complicated; legal counsel advising against the disclosure, and so on—there is no moral justification for allow-ing the family's anguish to continue.

In any event, the health professional's reaction to error will frequently be shaped by his or her learning and practice environments. If the individ-ual was trained in a patient-centered environment that insisted on disclo-sure as the only ethically right thing to do, the odds might tilt in favor of an ethically acceptable disclosure. If the individual's role models practiced deceit or dissimulation, however, then the likelihood of a truthful and re-sponsible disclosure of error may well diminish. Also, the degree of support and expertise the professional receives may influence the quality of his or her disclosure, especially if the physician's institution provides counseling, a careful investigation of what happened, a partner during the disclosure conversation, and follow-up support for everyone involved.[30]

The Perfectionist Fantasy

A great deal of literature discusses the perfectionist environment in which many health professionals of the previous generation were trained, as I discuss in chapter 5—instructors who "eat their young," embarrassing and humiliating students.[31] It is tempting to think that these learning environments may have been prompted by some sort of sadism or chronic hazing, but the pursuit of perfection seems perfused with a sadomasochism that assumes one must necessarily suffer on the road to Parnassus. If human beings are going to make mistakes regardless of how hard they try to avoid them, however, then a sadistic instructional response to students' errors will likely result in their learning how to better conceal or deny them. In any case, the natural response from human beings when they encounter a noxious stimulus is to make it stop, either by eliminating it or distancing themselves from it.[32] And because the encounter with error is a noxious, emotionally painful experience, many of us will unsurprisingly fail to seize the opportunity, do the right thing, and disclose.

In my 2005 book *Medical Errors and Medical Narcissism*, I attributed this failing to a narcissistic impulse, which I continue to believe is common in healthcare and in nearly all other professions: namely, the tendency of human beings to experience error as an acute blow to their fundamental belief in their personal adequacy or competence.[33] Error commission may trigger an individual's insecurities in the worst ways, because we are relational, interdependent, and communally engaged creatures. We fear that the commission of error signals our unreliability and inadequacies to others, which can result in our being rejected by a group we very much value. When it occurs among professionals, it's a disaster, because it can lead to license revocation, resulting in reputational and economic catastrophe. The irony is how an anxious concern over one's vulnerability to error becomes a formidable barrier to quality-improvement efforts. If we refuse to recognize error because we cannot bring ourselves to admit our vulnerability to it, then our patient safety efforts will be significantly compromised.

A contributing feature to these narcissistically based vulnerabilities is that one doesn't get into medical or nursing school by making lots of mistakes. For decades, successful entrants to such programs have finished at the top of their classes and scored extremely well on graduate school entrance exams. These students have learned that making mistakes must be avoided at all costs because errors spell career disappointment, not to mention letting down everyone who had faith in them succeeding. Consequently, developing intense anxieties about anything less than sterling performance as well as a near pathological self-absorption with achieving "perfection" is easy to understand. Not only is there no room for error in the evolution of this self-formation, but when errors do occur, these students are likely to react to them in unethical, psychologically dismissive, or unhealthy ways. Thus, if a significant challenge in patient safety is to develop a more tolerant and mature attitude toward error—marked by curiosity and steps toward enhancing error wisdom, improving hazard awareness, evolving techniques of constructive criticism, and making system improvements that are better able to absorb and learn from error shock—then that attitudinal change should probably begin well before students enter a clinical training program.[34] Alternatively, if succeeding in academically pressured environments means that errors trigger an acute loss of self-esteem bordering on self-loathing, students will be poorly prepared to deal with mistakes. If such an individual then finds him or herself in an environment that is equally unprepared to deal with the sequelae of serious error, we should not expect the interests of patient centeredness to be respected.

System 1 Performance: Automaticity

Patient safety scholar Ken Catchpole has written that "involuntary automaticity describes our ability to perform extremely complex tasks very quickly and with little effort because the relationship between stimulus and response is so familiar that it has become automatic, often short-cutting conscious analytical processing. The disadvantage is that it also means that humans cannot always avoid error by trying harder or consciously directing their attention towards performing (or not performing) a certain task."[16(p3)] So, when I was a little boy and did something clumsily, and my father yelled, "Be more careful!" or "Pay attention to what you're doing!" his words were for naught. Maybe for the next few minutes I would concentrate harder or go slower, but sooner rather than later, I would return to my usual, relatively automatic performance behaviors. As such, I behave like most persons. At least 95 percent of the time (if we are to believe cognitive scientists) we are on autopilot, executing cognitive-behavioral schemas automatically and with very little effortful thinking.[35]

This remarkable feature of our performative lives—that we are usually inattentively but successfully executing behaviors because we don't need to think hard about them—is exquisitely neuroevolved. Our brains are not designed to be hypervigilant or to pay self-conscious attention to every nanosecond of our conscious lives. Not only would our brains find this kind of mental focus exhausting, but being able to navigate our environments with minimal cognitive effort or automaticity leaves more energy available if something serious or threatening comes along.[36] Not having to anxiously scrutinize every conscious moment of one's existence enabled our Cro-Magnon ancestors to conserve energy better used to watch out for things that might harm them or take advantage of survival opportunities like hunting for food or fleeing from a predator. My brain is naturally lazy, but this laziness is designed for an energy-saving survival purpose.[37]

Consider how this can play out on a hospital unit. Physicians, nurses, and technicians are executing their routines of examining patients, writing orders, giving medications, performing interventions, documenting findings, checking off computerized lists, educating patients, and the like. Most of the time, they are on autopilot or semi-autopilot, having performed these tasks thousands of times. Yet, because their safety record is acceptable if not superlative, professionals regard their practice behaviors as entirely adequate. Nothing bad has thus far occurred, which reinforces their work habits, routines, levels of vigilance, and performance rhythms.[38]

When error-related disaster strikes, they are shocked. They do not recognize nor care to admit their automaticity because they never gave it much thought—which sounds like a bad pun but speaks to how automaticity works. When we drive our cars, for example, the vehicles transport us to work without our being able to remember anything from the time we leave our homes, get into our cars, turn on the ignition, navigate the trip, and saunter into our workspaces. Some neuroscientists speak of the "gappiness" of consciousness, referring to how we "fall asleep" for seconds at a time even while we're awake.[39(p198)] Excluding errors that are intentional—such as when clinical personnel do things "their way," which they know is contrary to clinical standards, institutional rules, or policies—many and perhaps most errors that cause harm occur unbeknownst to the error operator.[40] Furthermore, if our environments are themselves "pathogenic"—because of many sick patients or short staffing, unending interruptions, noise, new trainees, hunger, unreliable or new or unfamiliar technology, faulty communications, fatigue, new procedures, and seemingly unworkable policies—the likelihood of our avoiding error will decline.[41]

Consequently, when serious error occurs, a blame-and-punish approach is unreasonable unless the error was reckless or the individual has a history of error and seems untrainable.[42] To blame and penalize for error commission exhibits a misunderstanding of how human performance works. While the concept of "individual accountability" may sound noble, conscientious, and prima facie reasonable, its role in maintaining patient safety may be exaggerated because personnel are usually well trained and reliable in the first place. Individual rather than collective accountability for preventable adverse events will almost always be incorrect, as root cause analyses have consistently shown.[43(pp197-216)]

The ethical lesson of this is not to hold individuals less accountable, but to abandon the notion that humans can exert exquisite control (or mindfulness) over every second of their performance, and that this somehow justifies harsh penalties when they significantly err. Perhaps, too, the punishment mindset reflects the human tendency to want to hurt Nurse Betty if she has harmed a patient. Others' errors (although not our own) feel like betrayals of professional trust, which leadership can resolve by harming the wrongdoer. Also, Nurse Betty is an easy target because firing her gives the illusion that the matter has been taken care of, the system is now safer, and everyone can feel better. Yet, the systemic factors that enabled Betty's error will still be in place, lying in wait for the next harm opportunity to come along.

When an Apparent Error Isn't Error—When a Disavowed Error Is

An interesting corollary of the narcissistic theme I advanced in my previous book is how health professionals, especially physicians, will frequently but unjustifiably berate themselves over clinical situations they believe they mishandled. The irony is that many if not most of these situations—which typically involve challenging diagnoses, difficult judgment calls, or complex procedures—are beyond the cognitive or psychomotor capacity of the ordinary or prudent physician, and hence cannot be called errors or professional failures.

Nevertheless, the inclination of many physicians toward acute feelings of inadequacy about failure raises interesting questions. Granted, perhaps it is better that physicians do feel sadness or guilt when things don't turn out well, even if their feelings aren't justified or reasonable. After all, the physician who cavalierly dismisses an unfortunate incident as "just one of those things" might not have the kind of patient-centered sensibility that ethics prefers. Perhaps a dose of compulsiveness mixed with a more sensitive conscience is the ideal professional formation.

But if that physician is unreasonable about his or her fallibility and believes, for example, that he or she must make the correct diagnosis or choose the correct treatment plan on every occasion, then that physician likely harbors unreasonable self-expectations that blur the narcissistic line between ordinary and extraordinary skill. Just so, scholars have complained about how the treatment delivery model that continues to place overwhelming responsibility for patient outcomes and safety solely on the attending physician's shoulders constitutes an exaggerated sense of internal control locus that ignores the treatment *team's* contribution to safety. It bears repeating that twenty-first-century thinking about safety understands it as an emergent property of a collective. As Catchpole has written, "Doctors in particular take pride in the fallacy of being able to deliver high-quality care regardless of the state of the system around them, and openness can lead to negative recrimination by colleagues who are still entrapped by the mistaken view that only bad people make mistakes . . . [I]s it negligent that minor incidents are quickly forgotten, recurrent problems become accepted as the norm, and more serious events are rarely reported or learnt from?"[16(p3)]

The persistent but wrong belief that safety and quality outcomes result from individual heroics, rather than from collectives of vigilant people maintaining multiple eyes on the patient and on one another, enables error traps and quality pitfalls to endure. Consider an example from a team of researchers in Nottingham, who interviewed 80 physicians in 2007 on their attitudes to risk in perioperative settings:

> It was common for surgeons and anaesthetists to "tolerate" or endure certain levels of risk within the operating theatre. It appeared that suboptimal, uncertain or dangerous situations were passively accepted as normal features of clinical care. For example, we recorded how unfamiliarity with theatre layout or new devices, the late arrival of equipment, electrical disruptions to equipment, unprepared patients and inappropriately attired staff were frequently tolerated. Such situations present risks to patient safety, if only small, but for surgeons and anaesthetists, they were regarded as "everyday," "normal" or "insignificant" . . . [T]he tendency was for doctors to tacitly or passively tolerate and accept the risk, involving little or no acknowledgement or change in practice . . . This may be because such events do not in themselves require doctors to deviate from their normal practice, often being regarded as the responsibility of other staff members . . . By tolerating risks in this way, doctors normalize danger within their work, with potentially profound implications for organizational learning and the safety of patient care.[44(pS1:5)]

It seems perfectly correct to understand these physicians' risk perceptions as a manifestation of "me-centric" attitudes, because as long as the physician leader's schedule, routine, or role is unaffected, the patient safety threats may go unappreciated. Furthermore, when danger or a serious threat does materialize in the operating room, an individual rather than a collective model of recovery is frequently seen: the expectation is that the surgeon will innovate, improvise, "or modify established procedures in order to meet the unusual needs of patient care . . . [T]he expectation remained that coping with these situations rested with the individual."[44(pS1:7)]

The importance of clinical leadership is paradoxical within a group whose members have equal obligations to ensure that safety measures are respected. Safety measures are the responsibility of everyone regardless of rank. But if the line between clinical authority and patient safety authority is thin or vague, then system operators may assume others are responsible for safety measures.[25] But if we could rid ourselves of certain unhealthy narcissistic trappings of leadership, such as "I'm in control here and don't forget it," and transition to a team model that prides itself on maintaining multiple eyes on the patient and on containing the harm opportunities that are present, we will likely do better in reducing error frequency and severity.

Incident Reporting: The Gary Clezie Case

Recall that one of the strategies of mindfulness as well as vigilance is learning from the mistakes of others and from their remediation strategies. Incident reporting is an extremely important way to achieve such knowledge and insight, and in the years following the 1999 IOM report *To Err Is Human*, a rash of articles appeared in the patient safety literature on incident-reporting practices. The nature of and rationales for incident reporting are exquisitely reasonable and patient centered. In the ideal case, when a preventable adverse event occurs, an institution's incident-reporting system (IRS) generates a report of what happened that is forwarded to administrators, who investigate it. System changes presumably follow, and a report is made to some external body, "which aggregates and analyzes data from multiple sources and disseminates information broadly."[45(p1633)] When reporting systems work, their benefits seem obvious, given how such feedback information improves an institution's wisdom on reducing errors, containing hazards, and suggesting data-driven leadership interventions and safety strategies. But unfortunately, since their inception, these systems haven't worked nearly as well as they should or could have; and a case can be made that their less-than-stellar performance is a testimony to the maladaptive if not pathological reaction of health professionals and their institutions to confronting, confessing, detailing, and learning from errors. An example of IRS problems is the tragic case of Gary Clezie.

Case 7.1. Gary Clezie was admitted to the Yakima Regional Medical and Cardiac Center, in Washington, for routine outpatient shoulder surgery in 2009.[46] Things went terribly wrong, and two days following the surgery, the family agreed to remove the 47-year-old construction worker from life support, whereupon he expired. Investigative reports blamed Clezie's demise on nursing errors and the misadministration of pain medication. Yakima Regional, however, never reported his death or its circumstances to the Washington State Department of Health, the hospital's designated reporting site.

Presently, 27 states require hospitals to report various types of errors and adverse events, yet IRS problems begin with the wide variation in reporting requirements among systems.[47] For example, a hospital might be required to report to a state entity, like the Department of Health, or it might voluntarily report to an entity like the Institute for Safe Medication Practices or the National Quality Forum. It might also report to the Joint Commission, which accredits hospitals and can penalize them for not reporting. Adding to the confusion, some institutions question whether reporting provides any benefit, especially if the institution is distrustful about what the receiving organization does with the information. The reporting institution may also believe that reporting imposes a work responsibility that not only is unreimbursable but displaces staff from patient care.[47]

Problems only begin there, however, as the state-to-state reporting requirements differ on what must be reported and to whom. In 2009, Yakima Regional was required to report to the state's adverse event reporting office on 29 categories of adverse events, such as wrong-side surgeries, suicide, medication errors, abduction of a patient, sexual abuse, or a patient death resulting from the wrong use of a device (see "Adverse Events List," http://www.doh.wa.gov/Portals/1/Documents/Pubs/689003.pdf). Yakima Regional did not report Clezie's death to the adverse reporting center, however, because the hospital as well as Washington's Department of Health believed the circumstances of Clezie's death did not meet any of the 29 reporting categories. A report that circulated on the internet claimed that Clezie's nurses were supposed to have attached a blood-oxygen-level monitoring device to him following the surgery, which would have alerted the staff if his blood oxygen became dangerously low.[46] According to these reports, the monitoring device was never implemented, so when Clezie's blood oxygen saturation in fact fell to dangerously low levels, no one knew. Malpractice allegations claimed that this failure resulted in Clezie's suffering catastrophic brain damage. But failing to attach an oxygen monitoring device is not listed in the state's "Adverse Events List," such that his death could arguably go unreported if his demise indeed occurred for that reason. (Besides, one can also argue that Clezie's death actually resulted from his being detached from an artificial ventilator, which isn't listed among Washington's reportable events either.)

Another problem of the IRS is its failure to enforce reporting requirements. At the time of Clezie's death, only one person in the state of Washington operated the state-run adverse reporting center.[46] According to reports, she had no idea whether the state's facilities were complying with reporting requirements because it wasn't her job to investigate them. Furthermore, when error reports arrived, Washington, as well as some other states, didn't analyze the data nor did it provide any feedback to the individual hospitals in 2009.[46] But if no benefit or utility accrues to healthcare institutions from reporting, even though reporting requires (unreimbursed) staff time and can expose the institution to lawsuits, why do it?

State reporting centers are sometimes empowered to impose fines for not reporting reportable events, or they can even move to shut down an offending hospital.[46] But that hardly seems reasonable or desirable, especially for a facility like Yakima Regional, which is one of the largest hospitals in the state.

Another unsurprising reason that hospitals might resist reporting errors to external, nonconfidential sources is their fear of adverse litigation. In 2005, Joel Weissman and his colleagues from Massachusetts General Hospital and Harvard published a survey of more than 200 chief executive and chief operating officers from randomly selected hospitals.[47] These executives were from (1) two states that had mandatory reporting requirements with some of the findings being disclosed to the public; (2) two other states that had mandatory reporting whose results were not made public; and (3) two other states without mandatory systems. The data were collected in 2002–2003. One of Weissman's primary interests was learning what institutional leaders believed about the likelihood of lawsuits and overall patient safety stemming from error reporting and its public disclosure.

Weissman et al. found that, on average, 79 percent of respondents, regardless of their reporting requirements, thought that nonconfidential or public disclosure reporting systems would not only encourage lawsuits against their hospitals *but would discourage internal reporting of errors as well.* Their reasoning was that if no internal report is generated, then no external report would be generated either, thus diminishing the likelihood of being sued. And although half of the hospital executives thought that patients or families should be informed about harm-causing errors, many resisted the idea of their state's sharing error reports directly with the harmed patients or their families—a practice that I was unable to confirm happening anywhere in the United States. Rather than a formal arm of the state notifying patients or families of error, these executives thought that such information would and should be shared with harmed patients or their families by a facility's clinicians—an optimistic belief whose realization doesn't always happen.

Perhaps the most disturbing finding of Weissman and his colleagues' study is the degree of pessimism among respondents that reporting errors would benefit patient safety. Only 28 percent of respondents thought that reporting would have a positive effect, while 41 percent thought it would have no effect, and another 32 percent believed it would have a negative effect.[47]

Why would they believe reporting would not benefit safety? We've already come across one reason: that a fear of litigation might discourage internal error reporting, thus depriving the hospital of valuable data and positive system change. Another reason we've seen as well: if clinicians believe their reporting will result in little helpful information or feedback, they will be less inclined to report. Jonathan Benn and his colleagues found that if clinicians perceive their leadership apathetic and unresponsive to error reports, they will understand reporting to be without sufficient value and feel less likely to do it.[48]

Pessimism over the value of reporting errors occurs in other forms as well. For one, staff members will usually be focused on safety concerns that directly affect them: a pharmacist is unlikely to be interested in her hospital's radiologic error rate, while a pathologist will be disinterested in the hospital's fall rate. Consequently, generic error reporting centers could be replaced by specialty reporting entities, which has already occurred among centers like the Institute for Safe Medication Practices and its medication reporting program, US Pharmacopeia's Med MARX program, and the Centers for Disease Control and Prevention's National Nosocomial Infection Survey.[45(p1633)]

Also, clinicians may be confused about just what to report. Some mandatory reporting systems require information on an explicit list of categories, such as the 29 adverse events in Washington State or the Joint Commission's required reporting of sentinel events. Other especially nonmandatory incident-reporting systems may receive reports of near misses (where the error was intercepted before it reached the patient) or harmless hits (where the error reached the patient but caused no harm).[46] A 2008 study by Lauris Kaldjian and his colleagues found that only 3.8 percent of 338 physician respondents acknowledged ever reporting a major medical error, with about one-third of the veteran physician faculty and about half of medical residents claiming they didn't know how to report errors.[49] Also, the respondents admitted their confusion over whether to report a nonserious error, raising the question of how to estimate the gravity of mistakes. A medication error in one patient might be lethal, while the same medication mistake with another patient might cause little or no harm. Although it would be important to a hospital to learn how both patients received the wrong medicine, there may be considerable disagreement over whether to report the latter error.

Involving Patients and Families

A reluctance to involve patients and families in the safety process is well recognized, yet that reluctance not only continues, but their voices are absent even from postevent error analysis. I am reminded of the Josie King story, where Josie's mother's observations were dismissed by the treatment team, but the 2015 IOM report on diagnostic error offers another, more recent but sadly similar story:

> Sue's son, Cal, was born healthy in a large hospital, but jaundice appeared soon afterwards . . . Cal's father, Pat, and Sue were informed that treatment for such newborn jaundice isn't usually necessary. (Unfortunately, because of an incorrect entry of the family blood types into Cal's medical record, the hospital's clinicians had not recognized that a common blood incompatibility existed and could lead to serious elevations in Cal's bilirubin levels.) Within 36 hours, Cal's jaundice had deepened and spread from head to toe. Nevertheless, without measuring his bilirubin level, the hospital discharged Cal to home and provided Pat and Sue with reassuring information about jaundice . . . Four days later, Cal was more yellow, lethargic, and feeding poorly. His parents took him to a pediatrician, who noted the jaundice, still did not do a bilirubin test, and advised them to wait 24 more hours to see if Cal improved. The next day, at the request of his parents, Cal was admitted to the hospital, and a blood test showed that the bilirubin level in Cal's blood was dangerously high. Over the next few days while Cal was

in the hospital, Pat and Sue reported to staff that he was exhibiting worrisome new behaviors, such as a high-pitched cry, respiratory distress, increased muscle tone, and arching of the neck and back. They were told not to worry. Later it became clear that Cal was experiencing kernicterus, a preventable form of brain damage caused by high bilirubin levels in the blood of newborns. As a result, at age 20, Cal now has significant cerebral palsy, with spasticity of his trunk and limbs, marked impairment of his speech, difficulty aligning his eyes, and other difficulties.[50(pI.6)]

This case exhibits several factors that are known to lead to catastrophic outcomes. One is the way an "upstream" error—the incorrect entry of the family blood types—compromised the staff's perception of Cal's underlying problem. Perhaps the most persistent problem was the staff's anchoring bias, revealed in their customary understanding that jaundice in a newborn was usually nothing to worry about and their refusal to reconsider the care plan despite Cal's deteriorating condition. Sadly, the parents' concerns were dismissed as uninformed and needlessly anxious. Very likely, staff members were so confident in their judgment that they had become blind to what was actually going on with Cal.

Involving patients and families in maintaining safety remains a challenge for multiple reasons. As mentioned in chapter 2, some patients will not speak up for fear being labeled complaining, difficult, neurotic, or stupid, while health providers sometimes assume that patients have nothing to contribute to their care.[50(p4.14)] Many studies attest to physician prejudices or biases being triggered by a patient's gender, race, ethnicity, sexual orientation, age, mental health, drug and alcohol history, or obesity.[50(p4.17)] These biases might manifest among physicians in their dismissal of a patient's complaints, frequent interruptions, or orders for different treatments of the same condition in different patients, as Kevin A. Schulman and colleagues found in their 1999 study: physicians were significantly more likely to refer white men exhibiting signs of heart disease for cardiac catheterization than they were to refer black women with the same symptoms.[51]

Furthermore, patients can and will misdiagnose their symptoms—such as I did in 2008, thinking that I had a cervical radiculopathy instead of myasthenia gravis, which my neurologist correctly diagnosed in about four seconds. And yet, a patient's knowledge of his or her symptoms aided by a symptom checklist for this or that disease could be immensely valuable to the diagnostician and enable a more efficient examination and treatment course.[50(p4.19)] Contemporary thinking on patient involvement regards it as indispensable, not in the least because of the collateral benefits of good communications leading to better rapport, greater patient trust, and enhanced compliance. Furthermore, as the marketplace mentality has insinuated itself into our understanding of healthcare relationships, health professionals who dismiss their patients' voices are arguably violating each individual's right to be heard, regardless of whatever value may or may not reside in that recitation.[50(pp4.13-4.26)]

Consequently, medical training programs and contemporary healthcare delivery platforms insist on the involvement of patients and families. The IOM report on diagnostic errors declares, "Health care organizations will need to carefully consider whether their care delivery systems and processes fully support patient engagement and work to improve systems and processes that are oriented primarily toward meeting the needs of health care professionals rather than patients."[50(pp4.2)] Not surprisingly, the report recommends that health professionals improve their communication skills. I leave it to readers to peruse the voluminous literature on this topic, but what does merit mention is how organizations should commit themselves to pursuing educational programs that cultivate relational excellence among staff and their patients. Thus, institutions might emphasize the importance of understanding health literacy in their continuing medical education courses and lectures; they might insist that professionals use "teach-back" techniques that improve patient understanding; and they might invite representatives from local patient populations whose native language or culture can compromise their communications and interactions with health professionals.[52]

An important yet often neglected source of information for patients and families is print or audiovisual material on their ailments provided by their healthcare team. The IOM report also endorses patients having access to their medical records, an idea that some health professionals resist (just as they resist patients' audio recording conversations), but in a society that increasingly insists on information to the point of overload, that sort of access seems inevitable.[50(p4.25)] The OpenNotes initiative, where patients can view the notes recorded by healthcare professionals during a clinical visit, was warmly received by patients involved in the OpenNotes study, in which 70 to 80 percent of respondents claimed that they understood their care plans better and felt better prepared for clinical visits.[53] At the very least, patients and their insurers have paid for that data, so denying them access seems like

---

Box 7.1. Memorable Quotations on the Nature of Error, Diagnosis, and Clinical Reasoning

"An error is a deviation from the expected norm, regardless of whether it results in any harm."[4(p1402)]

"Medical diagnosis is essentially a special case of decision-making under conditions of uncertainty."[56(p553)]

"[A]nimals commonly make mistakes in the service of attempting to avoid bigger mistakes."[36(p476)]

"Physicians do not objectively, impartially identify and interpret features in a clinical case[;] instead, perception and interpretation are influenced by a hypothesis that is held in mind. This tendency to identify and interpret clinical features in light of a suggested diagnosis may lead to diagnostic errors through susceptibility to confirmation bias."[57(p527)]

"We all face a lifetime of vulnerability."[55(p721)]

"[B]ecause reliance on nonanalytical reasoning tends to increase with experience, it is possible that physicians with many years of clinical practice may be even more susceptible to availability bias than second-year residents, and this should be investigated."[58(p1202)]

"Physicians are slowly being convinced that fallibility is the human condition, and most readily acknowledge slips and lapses, but seasoned practitioners have lingering doubts that their own reasoning could be flawed . . . [R]estatement of compelling evidence has never been a sufficient force to change established clinician behavior . . . [C]hange may represent a midbrain event more than a cortical event."[59(p350)]

"Humans, quite simply, learn best by experiencing mistakes, understanding them and correcting them for themselves."[59(p353)]

---

a breach of contract. Concerns that patients may misinterpret their health information are easily countered by the opportunities that they have to correct their misunderstandings and the overall benefit of their being at least somewhat informed when they sit down with their physicians to discuss their symptoms.

Conclusion

In Lucian Leape's seminal 2002 article, he reported that barriers to error reporting involve time pressures, fear of punishment, shame, loss of rep-

"In health care, the premium placed on autonomy, the drive for productivity, and the economics of the system may lead to severe safety constraints and adverse medical events."[60(p757)]

"Experts are particularly prone to persevere with their initial ideas and to change their minds less frequently than would be ideal. Changing one's mind is unpleasant because it implies that the original thinking was incorrect."[61(p359)]

"[C]onfidence in one's judgment may merely indicate an unawareness of repeated mistakes. Bad judgment, like bad breath, is often not noticed by its source."[61(p359)]

"[T]he hardest problems to solve in medicine are the ones where no one recognizes that anything is wrong."[61(p360)]

"Physicians come to trust the fast and frugal decision strategies they typically use. These strategies succeed so reliably that physician[s] can become complacent; the failure rate is minimal and errors may not come to their attention for a variety of reasons. Physicians acknowledge that diagnostic error exists, but seem to believe that the likelihood of error is less than it really is. They believe that they personally are unlikely to make a mistake . . . They rarely seek out feedback, such as autopsies, that would clarify their tendency to err, and they tend not to participate in other exercises that would provide independent information on their diagnostic accuracy. They disregard guidelines for diagnosis and treatment. They tend to ignore decision-support tools, even when these are readily accessible and known to be valuable when used."[62(ppS18-S19)]

---

utation, anxieties over lawsuits, and a lack of perceived benefit.[45] These observations seem just as valid today as when Leape's article appeared—regarding errors generally, not just the reluctance to report them. It seems fair to say that despite at least 15 years of patient safety efforts, we have been less successful than we originally hoped in attaining the kind of error wisdom and patient safety practices that result in safer environments. But this only serves to remind us of how difficult these aspirations are to achieve, and certainly not for want of learning, training, good will, and commitment of healthcare professionals to their patients—none of whom (save for the rare criminal ones) want to harm their patients. Yet, as already noted, the failure of error reporting systems—which are commonly thought to capture only 10 percent of the preventable adverse events that should be reported—provides a lesson in the kinds of incentives or positive psychological factors that need to be in place.[54] Lucian Leape listed a good number of them back in 2002: institutions need to be less punitive, maintain confidentiality as much as possible, understand that preventable adverse events are nearly always the result of collective rather than individual fault, and practice a timely and expert response to error occurrence.[45] Perhaps the most challenging barrier to confronting and learning from error is its markedly threatening quality and, thus, our innate aversion to complying with it. Until we figure out ways to protect clinicians against their fears—such as by reforming the medical malpractice system so that health professionals will feel less exposed and by giving professionals certain tools to enable them to deal with their discomforts in ways that result in safer healthcare delivery—it is unlikely that much progress will occur.

In box 7.1, I've included several observations that I was particularly struck with as I researched this book. Just like the psychological challenges that attach to error disclosure, the purely cognitive ones that erode medical decision making will continue to plague us for decades to come. They reflect our all-too-human condition and the never-ending need to remind ourselves of our vulnerabilities and to take measures to reduce their impact on patient care. Perhaps clinicians, who tend to perform admirably if not heroically minute by minute, would perform even better if they would meditate on Croskerry's observation that "[w]e all face a lifetime of vulnerability."[55(p721)]

Interview with Fran Charney

Franchesca J. Charney, RN, BS, MSHA, CPHRM, CPHQ, CPSO, CPPS, DFASHRM, is the director of risk management for the American Society for Healthcare Risk Management (ASHRM) in Chicago. She has written numerous professional articles and has lectured or spoken for multiple organizations, including the Institute of Healthcare Improvement, the National Patient Safety Foundation (NPSF), the Hospital and Healthsystem Association of Pennsylvania (HAP), the ASHRM, the Department of Defense Medical Command, and the Commonwealth of Pennsylvania legislative committee for the 100,000 Lives Campaign.

Fran began her career in 1980 as a registered nurse working in the ICU, OR, and PACU of various hospitals in New Jersey and Pennsylvania. Her participation in the Pennsylvania Color of Safety initiative along with several other Pennsylvania hospitals won a HAP Innovation Award and a Patient Safety Achievement Award. She is currently on the faculty for the patient safety curriculum and TeamSTEPPS for ASHRM, and she completed a HRET Patient Safety Leadership Fellowship in 2009. She has served as director of educational programs for the Pennsylvania Patient Safety Authority and, prior to joining the American Hospital Association (AHA), as a member of the board of directors for ASHRM. In January 2015 she accepted the position of director of risk management for ASHRM.

Fran is an RN with a BS and a master's in healthcare administration. Her certifications include Certified Professional in Healthcare Risk Management (CPHRM), Certified Patient Safety Officer (CPSO), Certified Professional in Healthcare Quality (CPHQ), Certified Professional in Patient Safety (CPPS), and Distinguished Fellow of the American Society for Health Care Risk Management (DFASHRM). She has served as president of the Central PA Association of Health Care Risk Management, and she sat on the PA Medical Society Executive Council on Patient Advocacy, the Patient Safety Advisory Group, and the Committee for Quality and Care Management for HAP. Fran is an item writer for the CPPS certification and sits on the Expert Oversight Committee for the NPSF. She is also a certified trainer in Just Culture and a master trainer in TeamSTEPPS. She has acquired additional certificates in healthcare law, the ASHRM Barton and Patient Safety Curriculums, and Lean Six Sigma as well as earning a black belt.

The comments and opinions that Fran shares in this interview are hers and not necessarily those of the AHA or the ASHRM.

JB: Fran, good morning and thanks for taking the time to do this interview. So, we are stipulating at the outset that the views you express in this interview are yours and not necessarily those of the American Society for Health Care Risk Management?

FC: Correct. Nor are they the views of the American Hospital Association, which is the parent organization of ASHRM.

JB: Very good. So let me begin with some autobiographical things. You began professional life as a nurse, correct?

FC: Yes. For the majority of my years, I worked as a nurse in the operating room or the ICU.

JB: And how did you make your way into risk management?

FC: I wanted more control over my work-life balance, because as a surgical or ICU nurse, you're not in good control of your schedule—there were on-call obligations such as on weekends and holidays—and my family was growing. So I was looking for something more plannable or predictable for my lifestyle. I actually planned to transition into school nursing, and I got a position and even signed the contract. But when I told my boss I was leaving, he implored me to stay. Now, I absolutely loved what I did as a nurse, so leaving wasn't an easy decision. So, he told me that the hospital had an opening in risk management, and I said, "Why, I'm not even sure what that is. Don't risk managers show up when bad things happen?" But they thought I'd be good at it, and they asked me to consider it, and that's how I entered the field.

JB: Actually, my own story is not terribly different. I got a PhD in philosophy in 1976 and then failed to get a full-time job. The small college I was working at, running a federal program called Upward Bound, was starting a physician assistant program, and they wanted someone to teach medical ethics, so I volunteered. I don't think up until that time I had even read a bioethics article, so I just cobbled my first course together and read the articles along with the students. So, when did you start your career in risk management?

FC: Around 2000. Two things happened at that time: our hospital began to largely self-insure, and Pennsylvania passed patient safety legislation that required hospitals to report incidents, serious events, and infrastructure failures. The whole face of our hospital's risk management changed. It was a huge challenge to self-insure, so I learned a great deal about that. I had worked in that hospital for quite a few years, and I had extreme pride in our care and treatment. So learning about things going wrong surprised me. I mean we were a good organization, but we had our fair share of significant events. So I learned about those, and of course, around 2000 the patient safety movement was getting started. Now, most of the patient safety officers in Pennsylvania are risk managers, so the reporting requirements fell into our laps. And that created a golden opportunity for risk managers in Pennsylvania to move from a reactive to a proactive mode, which very much shaped my patient safety outlook and career.

I worked in that job until 2008, and then I was approached by the Pennsylvania [Patient] Safety Authority, which receives all the reports from the legislative mandate, to be the director of their patient safety programs. I accepted the offer and began working statewide. The majority of the reports we received were of near misses, where some problematic event reached the patient but usually didn't cause harm. But we also received what was termed "serious events," which were events that caused temporary or permanent harm or death.

JB: So, what did you do with these reports when you received them?

FC: The data were analyzed and aggregated, and then shared with reporting organizations. So, we would frequently find common areas that called for system improvement, and we'd produce a quarterly advisory report. We'd also publish deidentified case studies. One I remember was of a nurse who worked at two hospitals that used colored wristbands to convey important information. But at one hospital, a yellow band meant the patient was at serious risk for falls, while at the other hospital, it meant the patient was do-not-resuscitate. Well, the nurse confused the two and wound up failing to activate a resuscitation for a (fall-risk) patient she thought was DNR. So, we made suggestions for standardizing colors at Pennsylvania hospitals. We never set standards themselves because we didn't have that authority, but our staff would occasionally go to hospitals at their invitation and conduct root cause analyses, and failure mode effects analysis, which I'm confident advanced patient safety a good deal.

JB: So, you've been doing these things for 17 years and watching this field evolve. Talk about the big things you've seen in risk management during that time.

FC: I think the biggest thing is the enormous opportunity that risk management today has to be proactive. We need to be there before the big, bad, ugly things occur, and the blend today of quality improvement, patient safety, and risk management is perfect. What I've found is that while the quality department does a fine job, they are largely reactive, because by the time their quarterly quantitative measures (core measures, outcome and process measures) come out, the data are old, sometimes [by a] year or more. But risk management gets the calls, reports, or incident data right away, which gives risk management the advantage of responding to what's going on immediately and, hopefully, makes significant changes more quickly.

JB: Now, you've brought up a point that I've been acutely aware of since I started this book, and that is how QA, QI [quality improvement], risk management, patient safety, care transformation, even case management are becoming increasingly difficult to keep separate and how some hospitals have even absorbed risk management into the quality department. So, can you talk about the differences between these departments?

FC: Yes. It's the lens. Quality professionals are looking at quantitative data, core measures, which frequently come to them on a quarterly basis. The patient safety arm, on the other hand, is more sharp-end based, and they have the skills to identify patient safety events and look at system design. Patient safety isn't necessarily looking at the total enterprise system and discerning how one change can impact different areas. So, let's say there's a patient safety event involving labs and that a change is proposed that labs are now going to be drawn at 4 am instead of the current 6 am so that rounding physicians can have timelier results for rounding. But patient safety may not realize how that impacts the IT department for uploading result batches, or for integrating the lab system with the medical record system, or for printing and filing the results if they're still utilizing paper. So those "other" system-related issues may not be addressed if you only look through one lens. Risk management is different on the basis of its recording system. You not only can identify strategic things just in time but also areas for process improvement activities. So we don't have to wait for reams of data. Sometimes one report is enough to move forward. The beauty of linking quality, patient safety, and risk is that you can bring all those lenses together because, as individuals and individual departments, we have different skill sets and different ways of looking at things. To make that linkage work, though, you need to have a culture that values reporting. When I first started in risk management and hit the floor, people would scatter or ask, "What did we do? Why are you here?" But by the time I left that position, I'd have to allocate three hours to rounds because everyone was going to tell me about everything they're concerned about. And that's where you want to be. I remember our board saying, "Fran, what is happening? We used to have 100 reports and now we have 500 reports. Are we getting worse?" "No. We have become more aware of the risks." By the way and very importantly, we also get reports on "great catches." I have to admit, when I was a nurse, and I hung the wrong medicine, and at the very last second I caught it, I never reported that because I didn't appreciate all the things that had to go wrong in order for that to happen.

JB: Sure, you probably got that wrong drug from pharmacy. How did that happen?

FC: Right. Was it a prescribing error? Was it a transcription error? But I never thought about that until later.

JB: But if risk management got that incident report, they're going to be all over it. What about patient safety? Are they going to have a different approach to a problem like that?

FC: I think it gets fed through the system differently. Risk management can show the exposure of the event more easily and rapidly than patient safety or quality improvement, so the marriage among the three groups is totally necessary for the simple reason that they're stronger together than separate. So, safety will look at that from the perspective of the system design, but risk management can show the return on investment by making system changes. For example, suppose you had a medication error because of a transcribing error, and let's assume you had significant capital involved in your transcription technology. Risk management can go back and say, How many similar problems have we had? How many bad outcomes have we had? and attach dollar figures to those data. So, risk management is going to look at that not only as a system design issue but as a return on investment issue—assuming there is an investment—and hopefully how to mitigate the risk, make the system safer, and presumably increase return on investment.

JB: OK, so let's change gears. What do you think are the major patient safety challenges confronting health professionals today?

FC: It all comes down to culture and money. If you're not in a culture where patient safety is paramount, then it likely won't be paramount to the individual clinicians. We're all there to do a good job. Nobody goes into work saying, "Let's really mess up today." But if you don't have a culture that embraces safety, it may not be at the top of those priorities that you want to accomplish in your workday. If administration isn't paying attention to patient safety but rather to only increasing ambulatory access, where is your focus going to be? So, it speaks to the culture and leadership of that organization and to the competitive forces for achieving financial health. Of course, if you're not financially healthy, patient safety isn't going to matter because you're not going to be able to have patients.

JB: So, that leads into one of my most pressing questions: I want to ask whether or not we can cultivate an attitude of caution and especially foreseeability among our clinicians. So, they witness things on the unit that strike them as possibly dangerous, and maybe they make a mental note to themselves to watch out for that for their patients. But we know that in a lot of instances, they might not discuss that hazard with others, or it doesn't get up to leadership or supervision. And the other thing that makes this worrisome is the production pressures on our health professionals such that they don't step back and ask themselves wider-lens questions like "Is there anything bothering me about this patient's care? Am I missing anything? Why am I doing this?" So what are your thoughts on that? Do health professionals today have the time to be mindful about things?

FC: So, let's start with your individual practice. That practice has become honed and shaped over the years by experience. But if you're working in a culture of low expectations, where omissions and modest, nonharmful events happen often and nobody says anything, you come to normalize them, which can become harmful. Another thing we have to be very conscientious of is how we literally feel upon coming to work. We kind of think we put on a Superman or Wonder Woman outfit when we step into the facility as care providers, but if things aren't going well at home or you're not feeling well that day, it'll affect the care you give. Additionally, we have become extremely reliant on technology to assist our critical thinking. We had several systems in Pennsylvania that went to a terrific computerized system for predicting sepsis. The beauty of the system was that it was able to take key indicators from vital signs and labs and look at the predictability of this person going into sepsis, which is awesome. But what happens when that system goes down? Who becomes the critical thinker then? Because that's when you or I are going to be admitted; that's when it'll be down.

JB: Yeah, the Da Vinci machine isn't working, and the technician can't fix it. Now what do we do?

FC: So, while the technology is wonderful, it never replaces the individual's critical thinking: to be able to look at that lab value, the vital signs, the symptoms, and so on. So, the advancements are awesome, but I have concerns about what they do to our care delivery model. Think about patient records and charts. In the old days they were handwritten. You got a lot of information about risk issues, and I could tell a story about the patient from just looking at those notes. I could tell you that patient didn't get her medicine because her heart rate was too low; I could tell you that that drug was discontinued on Tuesday of her hospitalization. But now when I look into the EMR, I can't discern that story. With the handwritten note, I could get a sense of what the patient was like. Now, it's a bunch of checkboxes, which don't give me that sense of the patient. And some of it may be my age, but I think checkboxes are much different from a note or even a cut and paste, which have their own problems. So, I think we've lost some things, but I also think we've gained some things as well.

JB: So, as you look 5 or 10 years into the technology future, what are you seeing?

FC: Oh, the technology will be unstoppable. I was on a team on who should regulate technology devices. We downloaded this app that was supposed to do EKG readings for patients. The technology also allowed us to input the symptoms of a heart attack—shortness of breath, chest pain, nausea, sweating —and then we asked the computer what it thought, and it said "normal sinus rhythm." It never told me to go to the ER; it never told me call your doctor or call 911. So, a device like that might give patients a false sense of security. But I do think that things that plague us now won't plague us in the future. Frankly, I'm not sure what the future holds. On the one hand, the predictability power of technology is very encouraging. I can tell you that as a nurse in an ICU, my patient had every device to tell me everything. And yet, sometimes I'd know something was wrong when the device didn't. All the numbers were good, and the technology can be great. But the human component is so critical, and it's only through your experience that you know something isn't right. On the other hand, I'm really looking forward to the day when women can do their own Pap smears. But at the same time, when you're in with that physician, and you say to her, "You know, I just don't feel good," that opens a whole other conversation and exploration. The computerized data and analysis, even if it suggests a treatment plan, will ultimately require the physician to agree or disagree. Also, the interoperability of these systems is a must, and that hasn't been addressed yet. So, say I'm not feeling well while I'm traveling, and I have a chest x-ray for an upper respiratory infection. Don't repeat the x-ray when I get home and maybe still have symptoms, if it's not clinically indicated. Have the interoperability so that my physician can see the previous x-ray and make his or her clinical suggestions at that point.

JB: So, Fran, let me end by asking you this: From where you sit, as one of the leaders with the major risk-management organization in the United States, where do you see ASHRM's excitement about the kinds of initiatives going on?

FC: Well, we're on this journey now, and it won't ever end, because it doesn't have a finish line. I see the technology moving forward as very positive, despite its associated risks. In the future we are going to have interoperability. I just don't know that it's going to come fast enough for me. But the ability to share and streamline that information will enable us to give better care to patients and keep them healthier. You're going to see a change in health and health decision making. Early detectors like biomarkers are going to motivate prevention and early treatment. And I see the ability for risk management to be enterprise-wide and be able to have that oversight that will make a tremendous difference both to the organization and to the patient. Most importantly, we very much need to involve patients in their self-care and educate them about their choices and how best to make them.

I think we're in a much better place than when I first started in 2000, and I'm really proud of the advances we made. I'll tell you I never thought we'd do away with central line infections. I'm an ICU nurse, and those infections were virtually a guarantee in my day. And ventilator-associated pneumonias?— almost guaranteed for those patients ventilated for a long time. But many hospitals have gotten those rates virtually to zero. So it's amazing what we've been able to do as a collective.

JB: Fran, thanks so much. I enjoyed talking to you and listening to your enthusiasm and knowledge.

FC: My pleasure. Thanks for the opportunity.

8   The Standard of Care and Medical Malpractice Law as Ethical Achievement

[A clinician is] under a duty to use that degree of care and skill which is expected of a reasonably competent practitioner in the same class to which he belongs, acting in the same or similar circumstances.

Joseph H. King, quoting *Blair v. Eblen* (Ky. 1970)[1(p42)]

[J]urors are instructed to judge physicians not by the jury's sense of what is right, but by the custom that prevails in the profession.

Mark A. Hall[2(p126)]

Chapter Overview. This chapter begins with an argument that the plaintiff's burden of proof in a medical malpractice action is ultimately based in ethical principle, especially as it incorporates the idea of failing to comply with a reasonable duty that stands as an ethical (and legal) imperative. From there, it is a short step to discussing the standard of care, which is the content of that reasonable duty. The standard of care, however, is depicted as a moving target as well as given to multiple interpretations, so it is hardly surprising that it becomes a bone of contention in a medical malpractice suit—that is, did the defendants comply with the standard of care or not? The chapter ends with a lamentation that because so few cases actually conclude with a jury trial, and even fewer are appealed, the courts do not provide enough robust guidance in illuminating the extent or nature of the health professional's obligation. Nevertheless, the goal of the chapter is to make the case that medical malpractice constructs have important ethical dimensions, which gives the lie to the idea that law and ethics are contrasting disciplines.

The Plaintiff's Burden of Proof as an Ethical Construct

For a medical malpractice suit to proceed toward a judgment against the defendant health professional or his or her institution, a plaintiff must prove four things:

1. That the defendant was in a dutiful relationship to provide care to the plaintiff, meaning that the defendant had a professionally and legally recognized performance duty in the given situation.

2. That the defendant breached or failed to perform according to that duty of care—that he or she violated or departed from the applicable care standard(s).
3. That harm occurred to the plaintiff that could be measured or translated into some form of compensation, which is usually dollars.
4. That the harm occurring to the plaintiff could reasonably be thought to have been proximately caused by the defendant's negligent behavior.[1(p9)]

This burden of proof, which falls entirely on the entity making and advancing the legal complaint, can be ethically interpreted and understood in various ways. One interpretation is that it constitutes an instance of "wronging" in a medical context. Wronging as a component in a medical malpractice lawsuit requires not just harming someone but harming them from negligence or by departing from an obligation required by the standard(s) of care. Negligence is typically defined as a "failure to exercise that degree of care which a person of ordinary prudence (a reasonable man) would exercise under the same circumstances."[3(p309)] Notice, then, that negligence in the abstract doesn't require perpetrating harm, although it is often understood as failing in a recognized duty to protect an individual from an unreasonable risk of harm.[4(p169)] But for a plaintiff to succeed at trial, he or she must prove negligence that proximately (or more likely than not) caused a compensable harm.

How much of a departure from the dutiful standard is allowable may have varying degrees of latitude, but the standard itself will inevitably be determined by "professional services consistent with that objectively ascertained minimally acceptable level of competency he (the professional) may be expected to apply given the qualifications and level of expertise he holds himself out as possessing and given the circumstances of the particular case."[5(p273)] Ideally, then, the standard of care is central in informing the clinician's compliance duties.

Another way of interpreting wronging is that it constitutes an understanding of how consumers of healthcare should be protected. The protection they can expect is that their health professional not provide literally "sub-standard" care, that is, care that fails to conform to the prevailing standard. Patients cannot require that they not be harmed while undergoing care, but they most certainly can require (and therefore expect) that the professional treat them in a "reasonably" non-wronging way—a way that would comply with what a reasonable practitioner would do in similar circumstances in protecting a patient from unreasonable danger.[4(p169)]

Consequently, another ethical feature of medical malpractice is that it characterizes a minimally acceptable level of professional behavior by way of the "reasonable" person or practitioner.[4(pp173-75)] One component of a professional's identity is that he or she, through the execution of his or her professional role and its accompanying responsibilities, is inherently in a position to seriously harm a client. For this reason, humanities professors and hundreds of other professions are not licensed by the state, at least because their associated job functions do not anticipate the possibility of seriously harming others.[6] Thus, the foreseeable harm that could result from a health professional's negligence is vividly apparent and thus will not be socially condoned, at least in the alternative sense that any injured parties will have the right to a lawfully sanctioned hearing of whatever serious wrongs they allege to have suffered from negligence.

These passages may provoke anxiety among health professionals as they are reminded of care interventions that might go poorly and the seeming unreasonableness of their having to ensure that nothing goes amiss in providing care—which is impossible because healthcare provision is extremely complex and constantly witnesses mistakes, with unpredictable, non-negligent harms happening often. Yet, from an ethical perspective, nothing in any of the above paragraphs should strike us as ethically unreasonable or unfair. *Admitting the harm or threat potential in healthcare* is a feature of a mature and realistic attitude toward patient safety. Furthermore, requiring health professionals to make decisions and provide care that comply with their professional standards is at the ethical heart of what healthcare consumers should expect. It is ludicrous to think that as a matter of course, we should condone care that falls below a reasonable standard, unless the treatment conditions are such that it would be unreasonable to expect such behavior —such as providing emergency care on a battlefield with shells bursting all around or in a resource-impoverished environment that cannot maintain an adequate treatment infrastructure. What this discussion does provoke, however, is the fundamental and immensely interesting question of whether a particular professional behavior, judgment, or decision does *in fact* comply with the professional standard of care. Indeed, what do we even understand by the "standard of care"? How do we know and establish it? And how much leeway to depart from it should we allow practitioners before they face some kind of professional sanction or malpractice suit?

The Clinical Standard of Care: Three Characterizations

The legal tradition offers three ways in which the standard of care is traditionally understood.

The locality standard. For many years, this standard, which is also called the *community standard*, was widely used by states to determine the standard of care. Under this understanding, "reasonable" care, or the standard of care, referred to what the seeming majority of health professionals of a certain class or specialty practicing in a given geographic locality would do in a particular clinical situation or circumstance. To mount a defense in malpractice court, all a defendant health professional would presumably need to do is secure expert witnesses to testify that the defendant's conduct was typical, representative, or accepted according to what clinicians in that locale or community would likely do in the given situation. The locality approach to determining the standard of care was therefore something of a survey of the customary or "acceptable" practice in the relevant community of practitioners, which served as a proxy for the "reasonableness" of a given course of care or standard.[7]

The clinical practice guideline. While some states continue to use the locality rule for determining the standard of care, a more common characterization is the clinical practice guideline, defined as "systematically developed statements to assist practitioner and patient decisions about appropriate health care for specific clinical circumstances."[7(p1191)] Clinical practice guidelines are intended to suggest the preferred practice in a given situation, but as Chris Taylor has pointed out, they "may be developed using evidence-based methodology, or they may document common or customary practice, the opinions of an individual expert or the consensus of a group of experts."[5(p276)] The challenge that Taylor's observation raises is the quality of the justificatory basis for using such guidelines to evaluate a particular practitioner's conduct. That is, is the conduct, decision, or behavior justified according to a methodologically rigorous, multicenter, placebo-controlled, double-blinded brace of clinical trials? Or is the guideline established by observational studies or various kinds of case studies? Or did it derive from individual case reports and anecdotal experiences that physicians pass on to one another at conferences, in teaching rounds, or just by casual conversation?

The evidence-based guideline. A third candidate for discerning the standard of care is the evidence-based guideline. Here, the standard insists on the "best" evidence available because such evidence might have been poorly secured, such as from anecdote or subjective practice experience. The best evidence would be that generated by meta-analytic studies of the aggregated results (rather than the datasets) of well-conducted randomized clinical trials. Falling short of that, the next level of superior evidence would be discrete randomized trials with large, multicentered, double-blinded, placebo (or standard-of-care) controls that have survived enough peer review to appear in prestigious high-impact publications.[8] Less persuasive evidence would then include observational and cohort studies, case series, individual case reports, and clinical anecdotes. Care decisions and programs that comply with the best evidence should *ideally* be ethically and legally unimpeachable, because a medical practice or intervention resting on what experts consider the "best" evidence intuitively seems the best we can ask for.[2]

We have, then, at least three contending formulations of the standard of care—the locality standard, the clinical guideline, and the evidence-based guideline—each claiming a certain degree of justifiability or proof. Let's examine how well each one fares.

Problems with Standards of Care

The locality standard. If a health professional can show that his or her care complied with the given professional standard, then such a showing should have prima facie ethical as well as legal persuasiveness that it constitutes compliance with the professional's dutiful obligations and hence precludes the possibility of an adverse judgment in court. Nevertheless, the community, or locality, approach to sufficiently characterizing the standard has mostly, although not entirely, been dismissed.[7] Not only is the locality standard too subjective—as the practice variation from one physician to another, even in the same locality, could be enormous—but it flies in the face of contemporary healthcare education, where students are trained according to national standards, and where medical school, residency training, and board certification examinations are likewise nationally based. Furthermore, informational technologies make important scientific findings affecting clinical care available with a few computer key strokes, such that today's health professionals cannot plead ignorance of them as their counterparts could, many of whom practiced in isolated and poorly resourced environments, just a few decades ago.

Indeed, even if a particular practice is in wide use in a given locality, that doesn't mean it meets various reasonability criteria as a care standard: (1) Is the care being delivered consistent with the patient's symptoms or does it seem experimental, investigational, or just weird? (2) Is there some evidence available, such as an FDA approval, that indicates that the care being delivered is safe and reasonably effective? (3) Is the care being furnished largely for a patient's welfare or a professional's (especially economic) benefit? (4) Given that subjecting patients to unnecessary medical treatments may be dangerous, not to mention fraudulent, is the care being delivered reasonable in scope, intensity, and duration?[9] The Colorado Supreme Court made the point forcefully in its 1992 decision *United Blood Services v. Quintana*: "The standards of medical practice cannot be determined simply by counting how many physicians follow a particular practice. Negligence cannot be excused on the grounds that others practiced the same kind of negligence . . . ascertaining the objectively reasonable standard of care is more than just a factual finding of what all, most or even a 'respectable minority of physicians' do . . . In such cases, healthcare professionals may be held to an objective standard of reasonable care which differs from the community standard."[10(p32)]

Law professor Maxwell J. Mehlman also argues that alleging that a particular standard is the one in local use is a canard, even in the early days of the locality standard's popularity. Writing in 2012, Mehlman noted,

> Hardly any information exists about what physicians actually do. No one conducts surveys or polls to use as evidence in malpractice cases . . . Only five reported cases have referred to the use of empirical evidence of physician practice as bearing on the standard of care . . . [C]ourts in several cases have explicitly held that evidence of actual custom is not probative. Tennessee courts of appeals have twice rejected the standard of "what [a] majority of physicians in a community would consider to be reasonable medical care" as the standard of care in favor of "the reasonable degree of learning, skill, and experience that is ordinarily possessed by others of his profession."[7(pp1184-85)]

And I would be remiss in failing to note the pioneering work of Dartmouth physician and researcher John Wennberg, who embarrassed the locality standard's claim as a "reasonable" barometer of the standard of care by his findings that "[p]atients with back pain were 300 percent more likely to get surgery in Boise, Idaho, than in Manhattan. Doctors in hospitals affiliated with Harvard Medical School admitted patients to the intensive care unit four times more often than their colleagues at Yale University School of Medicine. Arthroscopic knee surgery—which would later be shown to be entirely ineffective at treating knee pain due to arthritis—was performed five times more often on arthritic patients in Miami than in Iowa City."[11(p34)]

The clinical practice guideline. In light of late twentieth-century medicine's frequent failure to substantiate common clinical practice with good evidence, clinical practice guidelines (also called "medical practice guidelines") entered the standard-of-care scene with considerable fanfare in the 1990s. Even so, such guidelines have also suffered from developmental problems. No person or group holds the mortgage on confirming the reliability of a practice guideline, as its development should be driven by quality evidence rather than someone's or some group's claim to authority. As practice guidelines have been developed, however, multiple guidelines often exist for treating common problems like back pain, obesity, or depression—physician Chris Taylor notes more than 500 guidelines for the treatment of hypertension and diabetes mellitus—and practice guidelines might contradict or be at odds with one another.[5(p279)] In 2012 Mehlman noted that the American College of Obstetricians and Gynecologists suggested diabetes screening for all women over age 45 every three years, while the US Preventive Services Task Force guidelines called for screening adults whose blood pressure was over 135/80 mmHg without recommending how often screening should take place. The American Diabetes Association called for all patients over age 45, particularly those who are obese, to be screened every three years.[7(p1212)]

Perhaps the most disturbing feature of clinical guideline development, however, are the conflicts of interest that many guideline developers exhibit, such as by serving as consultants or advisory board members, speaker bureau members, or equity owners in a company or organization that has a vested interest in connecting a guideline with a particular drug or device. This is a troubling finding, since "many of the newest ACC/AHA [American College of Cardiology/American Heart Association] guideline recommendations are based more on expert opinion than on clinical trial data."[12(p579)] Over the last 30 years, such conflicts have become commonplace because organizations that seek to develop guidelines will secure highly recognized persons in the relevant field of study, who, given their expertise, are likely to have economic relationships—for example, as a research grantee, scientific advisory board member, or stock owner—with some drug or device company. Ironically, but representative of twenty-first-century scientists, having a significant conflict of interest is for clinical researchers powerfully associated with having achieved significant fame or attention for their work.

Evidence-based practice. The obvious challenge is to inform and justify practice guidelines with the best evidence available. Not surprisingly, then, the evidence-based guideline has emerged as the summit of proof and justifiability because, as its name implies, such a guideline should be of optimal clinical utility and persuasiveness. If compliance with the guideline, however, results in poorer outcomes than those of less evidentially supported treatments, then something is clearly wrong with the science that advances the guideline.[13] On the other hand, "evidence based" might simply mean that the standard is based on the "best" evidence available, which is sometimes not good.[5] After all, the best evidence derives from well-conducted randomized trials, but they invariably require a sophisticated, elaborate, and usually expensive effort: The relevant hypotheses must be testable and their outcomes measurable, preferably in ways that can be compared with previous trials; research participants must be carefully screened, not only for the presence of the disease or ailment being studied but to ensure that they do not have comorbidities that can compromise findings; an adequate number of participants need to be enrolled, which is always a challenge and frequently requires an administrative team to maintain data systems and to ensure research milestones are met; data must be gathered and analyzed according to rigorous and well-accepted methodologies; and the findings must be gathered and interpreted so as to withstand critical scrutiny, both in peer-reviewed publications and in FDA investigations. Of course, nearly every aspect of the clinical trial must be vetted by an institutional review board, which will insist on compliance with federal rules and other regulations.[14]

Even a well-conducted randomized controlled trial can produce evidence that doesn't generalize to a large population of eventual users. The trial might have been not only conducted with a nonrepresentative sample, but also flawed by placebo effects, confirmation biases, low sample size, an unsound hypothesis, and so forth. Indeed, it isn't terribly unusual for drugs receiving FDA approval to fail in the marketplace, where continued evaluation shows them to be less effective than reported in clinical trials. In the 2013 study by Prasad et al., in which they surveyed 363 articles testing existing medical practices, published from 2001 to 2010 in the *New England Journal of Medicine*, the researchers reported that 146 articles found the practice being studied ineffective compared with a previous standard.[15] Another study, sponsored by *BMJ* and published as *Clinical Evidence*, reviewed 3,000 medical practices and found that "slightly more than a third of medical practices are effective or likely to be effective; 15% are harmful, unlikely to be beneficial, or a tradeoff between benefits and harms; and 50% are of unknown effectiveness."[16] Less frequently but perhaps more alarmingly, scandals have erupted over researchers withholding data on efficacy or side effects—such as in the notorious Vioxx case—only to witness significant patient harm once the drug was approved and consumed.[17]

Perhaps the most common problem with evidence-based guidelines representing the standard of care is the *specificity problem*. Whereas the problem just discussed concerns whether a research study will have findings generalizable to a large population of users who might be different from the control and experimental populations enrolled in a trial, the reverse problem for clinicians is deciding whether an evidence-based guideline applies for a given individual patient. Consider how patients vary by age, gender, severity of disease, risk factors, comorbidities, ethnicities, socioeconomic status, treatment variations (e.g., dose, duration of treatment, other medications), and geography.[18] Indeed, we would ethically condemn the physician who administered treatment according to an evidence-based guideline if he or she actually thought a patient's condition merited something else. Thus, Miriam Solomon, in her book *Making Medical Knowledge*, writes about the need for "domain expertise" in contrast to a "cookbook" style of medical decision making, for which evidence-based practice is frequently criticized.[18] The idea is that medical decision making requires a decisional loop between abstract knowledge gained from medical research and an ability to apply that knowledge to a unique person according to the clinician's intuition and personal experience.

Consider one more problem with evidence-based medicine that is especially vexing in a medical malpractice context: Suppose that a new treatment strategy consistently and inarguably witnesses superior outcomes compared with standards and treatment protocols that have been around for a long time. *How much time* do we give health professionals to adopt the newer standard and abandon older, inferior ones? At what point should an old standard of care give way to a new one such that professionals who have not updated their practice set might be guilty of negligence? How much "better" must the newer intervention be, and how do we measure "better" in order to fault and perhaps sue a health professional who fails to use it because he or she lacks the requisite familiarity with it?

The question is hardly an idle or an academic one. The fact that new drugs and devices are always in testing and being introduced to health professionals reveals a continuous learning curve for twenty-first-century health professionals. Their acclimation to new drugs, devices, and treatment protocols is never ending, while breakthroughs in genetically based technologies and interventions may, within the space of a few decades, make the delivery of healthcare in the West unrecognizable from what it is today. All these events pose problems for determining the standard of care, especially when it comes down to a real-life case that can materialize in malpractice court. Obviously, if health professionals are confused about the standard of care, they will be at a loss to effect compliance even if they want to.

A Hypothetical Case

In 2006, at the Clinical Congress of the American College of Surgeons, Demetrios Demetriades, Addison May, and Hugh Gamble presented a hypothetical case to the audience in the form of a mock trial.[19] Practicing trial attorneys were recruited as plaintiff and defense counsels to simulate what the evidential arguments might look like in an actual malpractice proceeding involving these circumstances (and remember, this case reflects the standard of care as it existed in 2006):

Admission to the hospital: A 22-year-old man suffers multiple gunshot wounds to the abdomen as an innocent bystander to a grocery store robbery. He is transferred to an academic Level I trauma center, where, among other interventions, he undergoes kidney removal, pancreaticoduodenectomy, choledochojejunostomy, and gastrojejunostomy reconstruction.

On postoperative day 8, a central venous catheter is placed in his right subclavian vein. A single lumen catheter that was not antibacterial or antibiotic impregnated was used with a Betadine solution for skin preparation. The area was covered with a standard 50 × 50 cm skin drape.

On postoperative day 12, the patient was showing signs of sepsis. The central line was removed, the tip was sent for culture, and vancomycin was started. A new line was inserted in the opposite subclavian vein. The resident wore sterile gloves and a mask and prepared the skin with Betadine. The nurse asked the physician if he would like to gown, wear a cap, and fully drape the patient. The resident said he didn't think it necessary. The sample culture came back with a finding of methicillin-resistant *Staphylococcus aureus*.

On postoperative day 19, the patient became septic, and his white cell count increased to 19,000/uL. Although central line cultures revealed *Candida albicans*, the line was left in place and treated with antibiotics because of a concern about inadequate future vein access and the need for ongoing parenteral nutrition.

On postoperative day 24, the central line was removed and a new femoral catheter was inserted. The patient failed to progress. Blood cultures continued to show *Candida* and vancomycin-resistant enterococci.

On postoperative day 32, a cardiac echocardiogram is ordered but not performed because of the unavailability of a cardiologist.

On postoperative day 34, the patient goes into septic shock, suffers a massive stroke, and dies a few hours later. Autopsy reveals embolic brain infarcts, infected endocarditis involving both sides of the heart, congested lungs, and a leak at the anastomosis of the Roux-en-Y. The cause of death is recorded as septic endocarditis.

Malpractice allegations: The patient's family brings suit, charging three standard-of-care violations:

1. At least three instances of negligent infection control occurred when the defendants (a) used a catheter that was not coated or impregnated with antibacterial or antibiotic agents, despite the patient's being at high risk for line sepsis, with the line expected to be in place for a prolonged period; (b) Betadine was used to prepare the skin rather than chlorhexidine skin antiseptic; (c) full barrier precautions were not used in inserting the central line—only a mask, gloves, and a small drape.
2. The patient's central line should have been removed on postoperative day 19, when *Candida* was isolated from the line culture.
3. An echocardiogram should have been performed well before day 34, especially when the patient failed to improve despite intensive antibiosis and was at high risk for developing endocarditis.

The attorney role-playing defendant's counsel counterargued that although the defendants did not use the best practices recommended by the CDC in 2002, the patient died from his wounds, not from standard-of-care failures. Defense experts testified that persons with the patient's kinds of wounds died 80 to 85 percent of the time. The defense also noted that (1) the CDC infection-control guidelines, which recommend the need for antiseptic or antibiotic-impregnated catheters, were used in fewer than 22 percent of ICUs a year before this event, which would have been in 2003; (2) a 2006 publication indicated that fewer than 30 percent of ICUs used full barrier precautions in placing central lines; and (3) an informal poll of 16 board-certified surgeons found that only 2 (12.5 percent) knew the difference between Betadine and chlorhexidine for skin preparation.[20] In summary, the defense's position was that the attending physicians used common treating strategies that were widely practiced in 2006.

Analysis

This is an interesting case as the plaintiff's mock allegations were based on the then relatively new 2002 CDC infection-control guidelines. The defense in turn tried to rebut those allegations by arguing that the CDC guidelines were *too new* and proceeded to argue that "these (newer) procedures cannot be considered standard of care if they are not widely practiced by the medical community."[19(p372)] Defense experts also argued that allowing the central line to remain in place and trying antibiotic therapy were not clinically unreasonable, especially as the patient was running out of central venous access, and that the newly implemented 80-hour week was to blame for the unavailability of a cardiologist and the failure to perform an echocardiogram.

A central problem this case presents is *how much time* society can allow health professionals, especially physicians, to implement nationally heralded guidelines such as those advanced by the CDC—especially the agency's Category IA recommendations, which plaintiffs argued should have been used. Moreover, although the case was published in 2006, the events of the case were described as having occurred in April 2004; the AHRQ report on the prevention of catheter-related infections was issued in July 2001, the CDC guidelines were published in August 2002. Consequently, because the patient received his (hypothetical) care at an academic medical center in 2004, the mock jury came down strongly in favor of the plaintiffs, believing that the education process at the trauma center was irresponsibly late. The mock jurors admitted that the judgment call on whether the central line should have been removed on postoperative day 19 was a tough one, but they also believed that when the infection hadn't cleared within an additional 48 hours, the catheter should have been removed.

Today, whether to remove the line would still be a controversial call. Non-antibacterial catheters are rare, however, and sending catheter tips for culture is rare as well (because it's hard to remove a catheter without contaminating it). Also, chlorhexidine has replaced Betadine.[21] So today, these details of the case wouldn't stand a chance.

The mock jury in this case found the defense's argument that the 80-hour work week prevented the timely diagnostic intervention of echocardiography entirely without merit—which they likely would today. To be licensed in the United States, any clinical facility would have to show it had adequate resources to meet whatever care needs its licensure requires. So, a resource failure in such a licensed facility, which would certainly be required to maintain sufficient numbers of personnel, seems frankly negligent.

Unfortunately, the resident's failure to use infection-control measures persists today as a problem for which physicians remain just as liable.[22] As would also likely be the case today, the mock jurors rejected defense counsel's argument that the patient died from his wounds, noting that the patient had, in fact, survived his initial injury, only to die weeks later from a potentially preventable line sepsis.

If certain lessons of this case are generalizable and can be compared with today's practices, they confirm the above arguments that the demands of the learning curve in healthcare are relentless and may often feel oppressive. But as Demetriades, May, and Gamble noted, "Physicians may be overwhelmed with work and might not think they have sufficient time to investigate current CDC guideline practices or implement these in their routine. But as demonstrated in the mock trial, if the hospital does not follow the CDC guidelines, it should monitor the CRBSI [catheter-related bloodstream infection] rate, communicate the infection rates to the physicians, and provide its rationale for not following the recommendations."[19(p374)]

While hindsight is inevitably 20/20 such that the patient's death highlighted inadequate infection control, a key consideration the mock jury made in justifying its decisions emphasized that the patient was receiving care at an academic health center, which was without a "reasonable" explanation for not integrating the CDC guidelines into its infection-control protocols. Although certain features of the case were perhaps clinically arguable or contentious, if hospital leadership was slow to adopt guidelines that came with powerful evidential support, then, as Demetriades, May, and Gamble argued, the institution should have been able to explain why. And if a convincing explanation wasn't forthcoming, then the hospital would become increasingly vulnerable to a lawsuit contending that a preventable adverse event occurred.

The Standard of Care: Noncompliance with Standard Operational Procedures

In addition to clinical standards of care, more general operational, or performative, standards of care are usually found in policy and procedural manuals that lay out rules, regulations, and practice standards. While clinical standards are relative to the treatment features of a specific patient's care, such as the correct dose of insulin to give to Mr. Baker, the latter are more generic, such as inspecting Mr. Baker's wristband to ensure he is the intended patient for the insulin injection. In either case, though, if a compliance expectation is written in the language of "should," "might consider," or "it is recommended that," a compliance failure will be more easily dismissed or forgiven than if the language of the statement employs words like "must," "will," or "is required to." Whereas the former statements are understood as guidelines—and allow the professional considerable discretion—the latter are standards, which are usually understood as constraining and, as Demetriades, May, and Gamble noted, require the professional to have very compelling reasons for noncompliance.

In my experience, noncompliance with relatively simple and well-recognized operational standards—especially the ones discussed in chapter 4, on the normalization of deviance—are just as if not more common in medical malpractice cases than ones illustrating noncompliance with clinical standards, such as those described in the hypothetical case above. Surprisingly often in malpractice proceedings, we are discussing not so much the subtleties of the best antibiotic to use (when they're all relatively good) or whether the patient should or shouldn't have had surgery versus a less invasive treatment, but rather failures to comply with basic rules like checking armbands, making timely and accurate notes, effecting good and timely communications, and ensuring that the patient's informed consent documentation has been properly completed or that the equipment works properly and is properly maintained.

James Reason has famously called certain system weaknesses or flaws "resident pathogens," because they tend to lurk within care delivery systems and are noticed only when disaster strikes.[23] What happens is that professionals become used to taking shortcuts or work-arounds, violating standard operating procedures, doing things their way, and failing to call attention to system vulnerabilities that they notice but that haven't (as yet) harmed anyone. Professionals are then lulled into a sense of complacency, relaxing their vigilance and becoming confident that the work environment is "safe enough." Studies have illustrated that when preventable and serious adverse events occur, they are usually due to multiple compliance failures coupled with inarguable errors or departures from standard-of-care requirements. For disasters to occur, as errorologists have been noting for decades now, these failures and their triggering error mechanisms must concatenate in a particular way to enable the materialization of a "disaster pathway."[24] Consider Case 2.3, in which the surgeon left a laparotomy pad in the patient's abdomen, the radiologist tried but failed to communicate to the surgeon his interpretation of the patient's scan, and the patient's sigmoid colon was damaged during the surgery. All three of these events needed to happen to cause the ensuing disaster. Such preventable adverse occurrences are proof positive that the system's usual defenses—such as practitioners' paying attention and remedying human or technological malfunctioning, completing tasks adequately and not skipping steps, and so on—have failed. At that point, one can only hope that the resulting harm can be swiftly remedied.

The Standard of Care as a Never-Ending Project

RAND behavioral scientist and lawyer Michael Greenberg has observed, "[S]tandards of care are evolutionary rather than static, and . . . providers have an obligation to stay abreast of new techniques and developments . . . [C]hanges [in medical knowledge] do not occur seamlessly, but by fits and starts, with the serial introduction of a multitude of new drugs, new devices, and new techniques, each of which starts out as an experimental agent with imperfectly known risks, and each of which involves a departure from what most physicians are doing, ex ante, in providing care for their patients."[25(pp424-25)]

The cases presented in previous chapters vividly corroborate Greenberg's observations. Recall that in Case 1.1 (sulfa allergy), the triggering error was the failure to upload the patient's drug allergy to the allergy drop-down box. Presumably, if her attending physician had seen the drug allergy listed there, he wouldn't have ordered Bactrim, and as he would later admit in his deposition, it should not have been ordered. Yet, was it error, indeed negligence, for the admitting nurse to have failed to note the patient's drug allergies from the documentation the patient provided on admission? Was it enough that the admitting nurse merely asked the patient for the information rather than examine the documents the patient had with her? And while we might be tempted to indict the nurse doing the history and physical for failing to transfer her knowledge of the allergy to the allergy drop-down box, she would later say in her deposition that she could not because the hospital's technology would not allow her to do so. The only way that the allergy information could be transferred to the allergy drop-down box would be by the hospital's usual data-entry process, which failed. Thus, the physician would later plead his innocence by saying that it wasn't his responsibility—that is, not within the standard of care applying to him—to ensure that any of that happened. But recall that his electronic signature appeared on the nurse's history and physical (H&P) of the patient, and that he had ordered a consult whose report noted the sulfa allergy. Does that mean that he, as the patient's attending physician, should have read these documents?

Somewhat like the case on infection-control failures in this chapter, this case also illustrates how a local standard—that is, "this is the way we've always done it"—can lead to disaster. Furthermore, this case sadly illustrates how an eccentric concatenation of events can allow error to evolve into a disaster: the failed upload of information to the proper place on the EMR; the patient's eventual and unfortunate need for an antibiotic—note that had she not begun developing bacteria, she'd have been discharged from the hospital, perhaps without incident; the physician's likely (and widely shared with other physicians') practice of not reading nurses' H&Ps; and his and a nurse's not explicitly asking patients about their drug allergies before ordering and administering medications.

The Failure of Medical Malpractice Courts to Illuminate the Standard of Care

For all the reasons enumerated in this chapter, and as law professor Mark Hall noted more than 25 years ago, jurors are the ultimate arbiters of the standard of care and whether it was followed.[26] Hall is in basic agreement with my position that reasonable compliance with the standard of care should protect defendants in medical malpractice cases, saying that "practice policies, if properly crafted, can have considerable defensive effect under existing law."[26(p126)] But he is also abundantly aware of the practical problems in assisting a jury to know and understand such a standard and whether it was properly implemented:

> The practical difficulties of proving just what is the prevailing medical custom break down this protective theory (i.e., compliance) in the real world. Lacking

any definitive pronouncement of custom, litigants must resort to the testimony of individual expert witnesses hired to evaluate the specifics of the case on an ad hoc basis; the opinions of the experts on each side are often in disagreement. When this happens, what in theory is supposed to be a process of comparing the defendant's conduct with established professional norms degenerates into a swearing contest. In this contest, in the view of many, when the plaintiff's witness states that the defendant's conduct was not within the standards of the profession, he really means only that he "would not have treated the patient that way."[26(p127)]

Thus, despite our contemporary age of evidence-based guidelines, defendants unsurprisingly will staunchly justify their conduct as having met the standard despite the plaintiff's arguments to the contrary. What the essays mentioned in this chapter by Mehlman, Prasad and colleagues, Taylor, and Hall collectively suggest is that the standard of care is in many instances widely acknowledged and practiced, but in many other clinical instances, it can be contentious, elusive, unstable, and, in the extreme, unknowable. Furthermore, because so many cases settle without a court's ruling on the evidence either side puts forward, the medical community is deprived of what could be important answers to important standard-of-care questions.[27] From the perspective of hoping for information that would either improve patient safety or at least better define professionals' obligations per those safety parameters, the ways malpractice courts disappoint that hope is lamentable.

Back to Ethics

As noted early in this book, the malpractice cases described in these pages suggest that ethical features of patient safety differ markedly from the kinds of ethical challenges that usually confront hospital ethicists and their committees. The latter mostly involve situations that are contextually complex, often owing to a curious mixture of rights and duties that interdigitate with imperfect clinical knowledge and system operations in bewildering ways. Certain rights claims may seem ambiguous or vague, such as responding to a 65-year-old woman's demand for in vitro fertilization, or whether to provide an organ transplant to a prisoner serving a long sentence for a heinous crime. These kinds of cases are ethically charged because they present themselves without conclusive or compelling precedents; they arouse marked and divergent feelings; and they continue to elude a consensual

settlement or agreement. Ultimately, institutions are left with having to develop their ethical policies and associated justifications in ways that seem to
best survive immediate ethical scrutiny and, then, the test of time.

In contrast, patient safety ethics requires a different model or approach.
As illustrated by the medical malpractice cases especially in the first two
chapters, aggrieved and angry parties must be able to show that (1) they had
a right grounded in a fiduciary or contractual agreement to receive care that
was shaped by a particular standard or set of standards, but that (2) this right
was disappointed in such a way that the plaintiff can convincingly argue
that he or she was both harmed and wronged. If the aggrieved party's argument proves successful, defendants will find themselves having to make
reparations for injuries the negligence caused. The ethical features of such
an arrangement therefore utilize a framework of dutiful performance coupled with liability for failure, rather than the kind of conceptual clarification
or analysis common to ethical deliberation.

The ethical implications of patient safety analysis for clinical practice
require cultivating the vigilant and mindful attitudes of health professionals who must commit to their patients' right to reasonably safe care. That
insistence requires the "twitchy vigilance" that James Reason described,
where staff are always conscious of if not preoccupied with the possibility
of things going wrong and implementing defensive strategies and practices
that are poised to prevent or mitigate any damage.[23(p241)] This kind of cognitive or epistemic orientation is not the deliberative analyses of the ethics
committee searching for a position that most persuasively resolves an institutional or patient care problem, but rather tokens an attitudinally and cognitively based commitment to patient-centered safety. That commitment
not only entails that staff rapidly respond to problems like technology or
equipment failures, untrained or incompetent professionals, poor informed
consent or documentation practices, confidentiality or privacy violations,
infection-control lapses and the like, but that they also mindfully self-mon-
itor their practice behaviors in ways that improve or at least maintain the
safeness of their environment and the adequacy and reliability of their skill
sets. Whereas medical ethics traditionally attempts to solve conceptual or
policy problems over what is the proper thing to do in a given case, patient
safety ethics targets the formation of an attentional and behavioral orientation that is anticipatory, self-monitoring, system conscious, humble, and
"feral." It is characterized by a chronic (but bearable) anxiety about which
assumptions, knowledge platforms, and clinical practices may be inade-

quate but are still (problematically) in use, and how treatment staff might be more encouraged to step back and direct positive measures and system-oriented improvement toward themselves and their work environments.

The Ethical Challenge of a Patient Safety Attitudinal Formation

Achieving reasonable safety levels in healthcare facilities is an inherently dynamic enterprise for the tautologous reason that the variables affecting it are never stable or static. Joseph McCannon and Donald M. Berwick have noted that patient safety requires "culture changes, new forms of teamwork, uncomfortable levels of transparency, disclosure, dialogue, changes in patterns of workflow, and constant vigilance at all levels."[28(p2222)] To add fuel to the fire, the roll-out of new, especially complex practices and their associated technologies is an optimal opportunity for failure, such as happened in the early days of HealthCare.gov. The 2015 IOM report on diagnostic errors describes how EMR technology has presented users with confusing user-technology interfaces, screens that are too congested with display clutter, and endless clicking, scrolling, and switching between a keyboard and a mouse, which can be enormously time consuming (with one study noting that a clinician could make 4,000 clicks in one 10-hour shift).[29(p5.10)] Also, rather remarkably, the design of many of these systems occurred in the absence of evidence-based studies on optimal user-to-machine interfaces.

The presence of balky or cumbersome technology that requires more system operator effort will annoy professionals who are beset with production quotas and productivity pressures, and virtually all of them are. Here is perhaps the fundamental ethical dilemma of patient safety, recalling the ancient platonic struggle between self-interest and duty. Just as self-interest can powerfully distract professionals from their ethical responsibilities, so production pressures can easily tempt them to omit safety practices or protocols that seem irrational, unproductive, pointless, and inefficient. As one nurse reported, "A nurse who takes longer to administer medications may be criticized, even if the additional time is attributable to safe practice habits and patient education. But a nurse who is able to handle a half-dozen new admissions in the course of a shift may be admired, and others may follow her example, even if dangerous shortcuts have been taken. Therein lies the problem. The rewards of at-risk behavior can become so common that perception of their risk fades or is believed to be justified."[23(pp92-93)] This kind of problem implicates the role of leadership in cultivating and maintaining patient safety ethics. For example, in a case with which I became familiar, a nurse was interrupted in the course of taking medications to a patient. The interruption was lengthy, and she proceeded to deliver the medication to the wrong patient, who experienced a serious adverse event. While the nurse later admitted she had not been following the five rights of medication delivery (i.e., right patient, medicine, dose, time, and route), other nurses on her unit confessed the same, and, indeed, their supervisors admitted not enforcing the rules.

Unfortunately, cost-constraint pressures represent a seemingly inevitable trade-off between patient safety and productivity, but the weightings of that balancing will fall to institutional leadership. The accompanying responsibilities are dizzying. Given that leadership must organize operations to maintain adequate revenue streams and optimize personnel and physical space, patient safety demands a culture of continuous improvement informed by evidence-based protocols; optimally integrated care with shared decision making among clinicians and their patients; constant monitoring of performance measures along with feedback mechanisms that maintain and improve performance; and, of course, maintenance of defense and safety mechanisms that favorably reduce error frequency and harm severity. We could also add to these leadership functions the maintenance of a "just culture," in which the very tempting impulse to blame and punish someone when things go wrong is restrained in favor of understanding how adversity happens, and multiple people and multiple systems are considered responsible rather than a single individual acting foolishly and recklessly.[30]

Consequently, an institutional identity that incorporates the patient safety sensibilities described here would begin with a collective and, admittedly, never-ending commitment to patient safety knowledge. Unlike the more traditional, contemplative approaches to ethics that are taught in ethics courses at colleges and universities, patient safety ethics would witness organizationally mediated safety improvements being doggedly and courageously pursued wherever they are needed. Unfortunately, the tasks involved in that effort are limitless and will, on occasion, outstrip the capacity of even the best, most safety-committed organizations. Thus, echoing an eminently realistic note, Reason has observed that "the only attainable safety goal is not zero accidents, but to strive to reach the zone of maximum practicable resistance and then remain there for as long as possible . . . An ideal culture is one that continues to drive an organization towards the resistant (or resilient) end of the (safety) space regardless of the commercial concerns of the current leadership. Three factors are seen to lie at the core of a safe culture: Commitment, competence and cognizance."[23(p285)] These thoughts recall the themes of the previous chapters: How production pressures compromise the safety practices and decision making of system operators; why education is essential, in terms of adopting operational practices that ensure or improve safety as well as (self-monitoring) education directed at personal skill development; and why, because human error is inevitable and ubiquitous, our attitudes toward its occurrence must change from shame and blame to learning and system transformation. These are all human challenges at deep and formative levels, such as social, formal and informal educational, institutional, administrative, research and knowledge development, and so forth, and they require infinite patience and respect toward well-meaning but imperfect human beings working in remarkable but imperfect environments.

Conclusion

We generally do not witness people who have been ethically harmed successfully prosecuting their grievances in court. Of course, one can sue for breaches of privacy and confidentiality, fraud, and defamation, but these cases are most commonly seen when plaintiffs feel they are able to convince the court that they have somehow been materially injured or harmed, such as by physically demonstrable suffering or by sustaining a loss of income or earning capacity. Of course, cases in genetics have appeared where health professionals either fail to inform family members of their genetic risks—an allegation that the health professional did not take sufficient steps to protect the plaintiff from a genetic risk that subsequently materialized—or allegedly inflict emotional distress in breaching a patient's confidentiality, where the patient had a genetic disease or syndrome that he or she wanted to keep confidential.[31] The overwhelming majority of medical malpractice cases, however, rest on the plaintiff's claim of physical or functional harm from the alleged negligence of a clinician. As discussed in my interview with Tommy Malone at the end of this chapter, these kinds of cases may be typical largely as a function of the award system in malpractice suits, in which plaintiff lawyers won't take cases where the projected damages are modest because the attorney's remuneration, based on the contingency fee he or she receives from the award the court allows, may not be worth the effort.

At any rate, the fundamental sensibility of medical malpractice actions—

where plaintiffs might receive some form of compensation for injuries they received from the negligent behavior of another who failed in his or her duty to act "reasonably"—constitutes the ground floor of protection from (noncriminal) wronging that Westerners have developed. Our ethical intuitions rebel at negligence-caused harms but assume other, less aggressive and explicit expressions when the wrong is "only" understood as a "moral" violation. Of course, without a demonstration of physical or economic harm, courts would be inundated with cases alleging moral slights, humiliations, disappointments, and grievances. Furthermore, personal injury lawyers would only have their imaginations and powers of persuasion to call on in requesting damages, as opposed to what they can more convincingly argue are damages based on lost wages, years of life, or clinically demonstrable pain and suffering.

This speaks to our contemporary culture's divergent sensibilities over what persons are formally owed for alleged harms that are independent of physical or economic loss. Our major moral progress has seemingly been in instances of civil rights, where courts and legislatures have insisted that persons be entitled by law to certain socioeconomic opportunities, benefits, and rights of access. For much of the rest, and despite Kant's requiring us to treat one another as ends and not merely as means, we are at odds over interpreting and implementing his meaning of "the person as an end in him or herself." We have consensually agreed that people should not be raped or unreasonably harassed, but we are less certain about their rights to access healthcare, and not at all agreed about what a right to a decent minimum of welfare entails by way of a legislative response.

Such disagreements, however, ultimately define and distinguish cultures from one another and are what historians and ethnographers study and write about. Although courts will continue to see new and imaginative causes of action that aggrieved plaintiffs advance, recent history suggests that we will more likely see rather unpredictable contractions and expansions in what we can morally require from one another, especially by way of personal freedoms, rights to government-sponsored welfare and education programs, and the content of a decent standard of living. But these latter considerations are beyond the scope of this book. Fortunately, matters bearing on patient safety are more accessible, or at least seem to call on if not more consensually shared beliefs and values, then at least ones that can be operationalized by our healthcare and legal systems. There is an old ethical adage that "ought implies can." Both law and ethics, therefore, need to develop characterizations or visions of healthcare work that are reasonable, so that clinicians can perform safely, effectively, and ethically.

An Interview with Tommy Malone

Thomas Malone is the founder of Malone Law in Atlanta, Georgia. He is a past president of the American Board of Professional Liability Attorneys, the official certifying body sanctioned by the American Bar Association for certification of competency in handling professional negligence cases. He is a member of *Best Lawyers*, the oldest peer-review publication in the legal profession, as well as Super Lawyers, a listing of attorneys from more than 70 practice areas who have attained a high degree of peer recognition and professional achievement. He has been named a member of the Bar Register of Preeminent Lawyers with Martindale-Hubbell, a listing of law practices that have earned the highest rating in the Martindale-Hubbell Law Directory and have been designated by their colleagues as preeminent in their field. He is a fellow of the Litigation Counsel of America, an invitation-only trial lawyer honorary society composed of less than one-half of one percent of American lawyers. Fellows are selected based on effectiveness and accomplishment in litigation, at both the trial and the appellate levels, and superior ethical reputation. For more than 40 years, he has litigated cases involving catastrophic personal injury and wrongful death, and has obtained a multitude of jury verdicts in excess of $1 million, including one in excess of $49 million.

JB: Tommy, how does the right of a patient to recover in a court of law for injuries caused by medical malpractice contribute to patient safety?

TM: First, we should define medical negligence. Medical negligence that results in harm to the patient is what's at the center of a medical malpractice claim. Medical malpractice occurs when the physician or the healthcare provider fails to exercise that degree of care, skill, and diligence that is ordinarily exercised by members of the same profession or same specialty under like or similar conditions and like surrounding circumstances. That departure is what we must prove in any medical negligence case. We must prove the physician didn't comport with that degree of care, skill, and diligence that is ordinarily exercised, and we must also prove harm resulted from that departure. I should mention here that the harm must be significant in order for any claim to be brought. These claims are very time consuming and very expensive. No lawyer can afford to take on a case involving a small or insignificant injury no matter how clear the carelessness.

So, the primary goal of the medical malpractice case is to realize some kind of monetary award, whether by a settlement or a jury verdict, for the plaintiff. I was talking to a physician last night, and I asked him what he thought about the medical malpractice system, and he said, "None of us like it, but we know it has to exist."

JB: OK and spoken like a litigator. But we do know that one of the collateral benefits of the medical malpractice system is that a claim may cause a hospital or a professional to examine their practices and change some behaviors or policies that may have caused that adversity to occur. I mean, you must have seen that in your career?

TM: Oh sure, and I can tell you a story from a case I recently handled. The case involved a patient who had gone in for a prostatectomy. Sometime after the surgery, a senior urologic fellow comes in to check on him, and she's focused on the surgical site, which is literally her specialty area. The patient is lying in bed, and he's saying, "I'm having trouble breathing, and I've got a feeling of fullness in my stomach." The urology fellow somewhat impatiently says, "You need to get up and walk around. That'll get rid of your complaints." The physician raises the head of his bed and tells him to get up and walk over to a chair in his room. He says, "OK, I'll try." The physician walks out of the room, but the patient, who has gotten up and walked over to the chair and sits down, says to his wife, "Get the doctor, I'm really having trouble breathing." She goes out into the hall and when she and a doctor return, the patient has fallen out of the chair. He's on the floor, aspirating, and is virtually unconscious. Two days later, he dies in the ICU. Now, what that hospital subsequently did was to create a video with my client telling her story. All the physicians watched, and that reminds them to examine the entire patient, not just their specialty area. So, not only might that video instruction prevent another incident like that one from happening, but it gave my client solace in knowing that her husband's life wasn't swept under the table.

JB: How has the standard of care figured in your career and in your strategy as a litigator? When you hire an expert witness, are you looking more at his or her believability as an expert or his or her ability to quote the clinical literature or what? And again, I'm wanting to focus on how you strategically handle the standard-of-care issue as the litigation proceeds.

TM: Well, we get between 800 and 1,000 medical calls a year. We take about 20 cases. We screen these cases on two points: one is the damages; the other is the carelessness. The higher the likely damages are, the closer we're going to look at the carelessness. The truth is that no lawyer today can take on a medical negligence case only worth $100,000. If they do, they won't be doing it for long. Frankly, we have to be prepared to spend whatever it takes. For example, in birth injury cases, a common defense tactic is to create confusion over causation, in other words, arguing that the injury could have been due to various kinds of things, not necessarily negligence. That means we'll often have to get experts in every one of those fields to refute those testimonies, and that will run up our expenses significantly. In fact, in the last birth injury case we tried, which we had to try twice, we had over $500,000 in expenses.

And yet I can tell you that most of my clients are not in it for the money unless they need the money to care for their loved one. All of them want to make sure that this doesn't happen to somebody else.

JB: And this also speaks to the need for families to get closure. So, granted that there has to be sufficient damages for you to take a case, that degree or magnitude of departure from the standard of care is clearly going to be a deciding factor.

TM: Sure, how provable it is. How clear it is. And there's also the challenge we have in dealing with inaccurate impressions or assumptions of the lay public. For example, if someone said, "I'm going in to have my appendix out, or my gall bladder removed, or I'm going in to have a baby," all their friends and loved ones will say, "Well, I'll see you next week." But if you say, "I'm going in to have a brain tumor removed," even if it's a superficial tumor, everybody says, "I'll pray for you." So, a simple craniotomy to excise a lesion on the outside will be a tougher case to win than an appendectomy that goes bad.

You asked about what I look for in an expert. The first is that he or she must be credentialed or board certified. Georgia even has a law that your medical expert must have practiced or taught three out of the last five years with sufficient frequency on the matter being litigated. And that's not a bad part of the tort reform movement because you want a top expert. But I always tell my experts, I don't want you stretching anything to make a case here. You do me no favor in trying to make a case where none exists.

JB: So, the expert witness is essentially or ideally there to represent the standard of care.

TM: Yes, standard-of-care opinion is required as is causation testimony. Because it's a matter of opinion, the standards can be subject to variance. But I don't want one of my experts thinking there "might" be a deviation from the standard of care but then telling me, "Oh, it's a clear departure." They don't do me a favor by doing that. And in a way, that's why screening is the key to successful plaintiff work. If you take every case that comes along, you're going to go broke very quickly.

JB: So, my impression is that doctors typically hate the whole med mal platform in the United States, while only the more serious ones have advocated alternatives like no fault. This isn't going to make me any friends among physicians, but in the almost 40 years I've been professionally observing them, I don't think there's any question that some of them, maybe the majority of them, believe that the profession deserves some special consideration so that when they err, they should just get a pass. Just forget about it or at least let the doctor go on doing good things for patients. On the other hand, if you just bought a new lawn mower and it blows up in your face when you try to start it, nobody is going to criticize your right to recover damages from the manufacturer.

TM: When doctors get up in the morning and they head off to work, they know they're doing God's work, and they don't intend to hurt anybody. So when they do hurt somebody because they're careless, they think they should get some kind of special consideration because they didn't mean to hurt anybody. Well, that's true of every segment of our society. Think about the preacher who loads up his car with clothes for the homeless, and he's going down the road looking for the homeless and doesn't see the stop sign and runs over somebody in the middle of the road and paralyzes them. He didn't mean to do it, and he's doing God's work.

JB: Tommy, I've had cases where the physician's or nurse's denial that they violated the standard of care has been mind boggling. I mean, what to any person would seem a clear-cut case of negligence is staunchly denied by the defendant. If I was a plaintiff lawyer, that would drive me crazy.

TM: Well, you have to remember that they have a lawyer telling them they didn't violate the standard of care, and that's why they are defending the case.

JB: So, if they're defending, they have to have that bunker mentality.

TM: Yes, and I think it comes from their defense lawyers because they want their defendants to believe that they did nothing wrong. It's not going to help defendants to get on the stand with them thinking they did something wrong.

Until discovery is complete, they cannot know for sure whether the case is defensible.

JB: Tommy, there was a study that came out about 6 months ago that showed that physicians who practice defensive medicine were sued five times less frequently than physicians who are more conservative and more reasonable.

TM: Well, it's easy to believe that, but it may be more complicated from the clinical side. A few years ago, I gave a talk, and I asked the audience, "How many of you believe in defensive medicine?" and a lot of people raised their hands. And I asked, "How many of you realize that practicing defensive medicine on a Medicare or Medicaid patient is committing fraud?" Because if you order the test that is not for the benefit of the patient but is for the benefit of the doctor, that's Medicare fraud. But here's the thing: I don't think any reasonable doctor practices defensive medicine. If there was any reasonable basis whatsoever for ordering the test, wouldn't you want it for yourself or your loved one? And wouldn't the doctor want to order it? So, I'd change the adjectives and call it careful medicine. Why would a doctor order a test that had no potential benefit for the patient?

JB: Well, patients obviously like it, too, when the physician says, "We're not going to leave any stone unturned here." So, patients feel that they're getting the Cadillac treatment.

TM: But I think that's good medicine if there's a basis for those tests. Doctors have been taught to think of it in terms of defensive, but I can't think that a physician orders any test or study that doesn't have a meaningful benefit for the patient—unless, like I said, he doesn't care about committing fraud.

JB: The interesting question is the probability or frequency of that benefit: Should it be beneficial for one in ten patients, one in a hundred, one in a thousand?

TM: I would say whenever the potential benefit outweighs the risk, then it's reasonable to order the test.

JB: So, what advice, based on your decades of experience in trying cases and seeing negligence going down, what advice would you give to health professionals?

TM: I'd tell them to slow down. In so many of our cases, the nurses and doctors are working too fast and ignoring things that they should be paying attention to.

JB: Tommy, is there anything else you'd like to add?

TM: Well, maybe this is more advice for lawyers than health professionals, but I think defense lawyers should realize that when they consider settling a case, they're going to need to do all their discovery first. Because they would be enlightened by the discovery, and their decisions about whether or not to move forward would be better informed.

JB: So, I always thought that the defense bar wants to draw out discovery, not only to bill their clients, but especially to see what you have.

TM: But seeing what we have is more like seeing whether or not we caught you. But they should be able to find out from their side whether the case ought to be settled.

JB: I think we're done. Thanks, Tommy.

TM: You're welcome.

9 The Present and the Future

Me to a long-time and very experienced plumber: "George, when do you
know that a job is going to be difficult?"

George: "Before I start."

Chapter Overview. This chapter recalls certain themes from preceding ones but places them in light of twenty-first-century neuroscience.
The stark problem is how difficult it is for humans to realize the aspirations of vigilance, mindfulness, compliance, and humility given that the
human nervous system has remained relatively unchanged structurally for
the last 30,000 years. The chapter ends with a reflection on the inexorability of change, especially technological change, and with an interview with
Dr. Bob Wachter, a patient safety expert who coined the term "hospitalist."

Patient Safety and the Human Brain

Consider how the world of patient safety has changed. We have progressed
from early twentieth-century clinical environments that had only begun
to appreciate the value of sterile technique and were yet without antibiotics or standardized medical or nursing training, to our present-day healthcare environments, which are unable to function without them. But the
twentieth-century game changer for patient safety, I would argue, was
James Reason's (and others') discovery of the evolution of disasters—which
begin as multiple, discrete, seemingly unrelated, and often hardly notice-
able errors, mishaps, or deviations from care standards, but with the assistance of other unpredictable variables (e.g., unwarranted assumptions, poor
judgment calls, system operator fatigue, epistemic unfamiliarity or failure,
etc.) coalesce into a harm pathway that ends in disaster.

Reason's "swiss cheese" model was patient safety's paradigm shift, similar to what Einstein's relativity theory, Copernicus's heliocentric theory,
and Hippocrates's naturalism were to science. We are still absorbing the
model's ethical lessons: that humans are naturally error prone; that degraded systems are indispensable in causing iatrogenic catastrophes; that
instead of blaming people for errors, we should be admitting, investigating,

and remediating our error traps and pitfalls; that replacing humans with machines will largely result in safer environments, but in all likelihood will create new safety challenges; that transparency and teamwork are better patient safety strategies than concealment and oppressive leadership hierarchies; and that innovation will demand that system operators exercise vigilance, mindfulness, compliance, and humility throughout their careers.

Despite the changes wrought by innovation, however, one thing that hasn't changed in the last 30,000 years is the morphology and neurophysiology of the human brain and its immense reliance on unconscious, limbic operations for most of its cognitive and psychomotor functioning. Hart Blanton and others have looked to evolution for an explanation of the ubiquity and omnipresence of System 1 "thinking" and opine that we have neurologically evolved to make rapid decisions and discriminations that resolve most of our navigational problems with only occasional, modest error.[1] Evolution has equipped us with neural networks that make far more correct decisions than incorrect ones, as well as more lesser-magnitude errors than greater-magnitude ones. But that's only reasonable: if our species persistently made highly injurious errors with great frequency, we would have become extinct long ago.

Nevertheless, our neural architecture is one of the patient safety bugaboos with which we will always wrestle. Humans are magnificently adaptive creatures, and our personal survival interests are paramount. So we continue to seek the most efficient and least burdensome work strategies to accomplish our tasks, even if they sometimes seem to require deviations from policies, regulations, and standards. Our hazard imaginations (or foreseeability) are very limited, and it sometimes takes years of experience to know when one is unprepared to undertake a task or to simply appreciate a task's complexity and where the challenges lie. Thus, my wise and experienced plumber, George, told me that his four decades of experience enabled him to recognize a tough job before he began it. He also told me that when he was a young apprentice, it took him eighteen attempts to fix one of his client's plumbing problems—a humiliating experience to be sure, but if mistakes are one of our best teachers, George probably learned a ton of valuable lessons from that job.

Unlike plumbing, though, where the professional may have only himself to blame for repair failures, the disaster pathways that this book describes usually have multiple operators laying the "asphalt" that paves the way for disaster. And unless one has training in "catastrophology," where the role of multiple people making multiple mistakes is axiomatic, our primitive lizard brains will be very tempted to blame and prosecute whomever we can—except ourselves, to whom we are exquisitely empathic. Our natural urge is to expel the more salient error perpetrators from our midst (e.g., the nurse who gives the patient the wrong medication), because his or her very presence creates noxious feelings among us that we want stopped.

Improving patient safety therefore requires the difficult job of ridding ourselves of these lizard brain biases and inclinations, giving up the illusion of perfection, and buckling down to learning and absorbing patient safety knowledge. Serious error commission is sobering and shocking. Our self-esteem-based need to believe that we are competent navigators of our environments is destabilized by serious error, and the accompanying feeling that we cannot trust our performance is terribly unsettling. Little prepares one for it, unless he or she is carefully trained to appreciate how systems fail, where likely failure pockets reside, what the prelude to disaster feels like, and how one might effect a recovery from imminent disaster or at least diminish an error's destructive potential.

That training in patient safety comes late in clinical curricula is lamentable but perhaps understandable. I suspect that most healthcare students learn about errors and the harms they cause from on-the-job experiences or at lectures specifically devoted to discrete safety issues like infection control, fall prevention, and safe medication delivery. And while most of my medical students, whom I see in their third year of training, have heard of the swiss cheese model of disaster, I know that they are often unprepared to differentiate an error from a complication, that they constantly announce an interest in error disclosure training, and that they often report witnessing errors being disclosed very poorly or at least in a less than patient-centered way. To be fair, though, they often report witnessing ethically above-board error disclosures.

My impression from studying patient safety scholarship and attending conferences over the years is that healthcare delivery systems have fallen disappointingly short of the hoped-for error reduction targets originally set in 2000, although certain safety parameters, like reducing ventilator-acquired pneumonias, have greatly declined in many hospitals. Still, health professionals are hesitant to purchase and integrate new technologies into their clinical practices that might reduce errors; administrators continue to oppress clinicians with patient loads that exceed their capacity to deliver care safely; and changes to care standards brought on by new drugs and devices continue apace but also create relentless learning demands on the workforce. And while younger health professionals can probably meet these intellectual and psychomotor challenges better than their older counterparts, the fact that the average age of today's floor nurse is around 50 should give us patient safety pause.[2]

Furthermore, corrective responses to error often seem to be determined by the gravity of harm that eventuates. Because a serious harm-causing error is often glaringly obvious, it may receive considerable attention from risk management and sometimes, such as in the sexual attack case described in chapter 2, witness remedial measures, like architectural changes to the unit, almost immediately. But if an error causes no harm, which is true of the majority, these mistakes will often receive no serious attention, so that their causal factors, or what Reason calls the system's "resident pathogens," remain on the floor, waiting for the next opportunity to strike.

An interesting thing to contemplate is how these "pathogens" will intersect with the onslaught of health information that will be made available from twenty-first-century technologies. Certainly, humans living in the near future will have access to immense databases whose technologies monitor and report on their health and welfare. Siddhartha Mukherjee recently wrote, "Our cell phones [of the future] would analyze shifting speech patterns to diagnose Alzheimer's. A steering wheel would pick up incipient Parkinson's through small hesitations and tremors. A bathtub would perform sequential scans as you bathe, via harmless ultra-sound or magnetic resonance, to determine whether there's a new mass in an ovary that requires investigation . . . [W]e would shuttle from the grasp of one algorithm to the next."[3(p51)]

The challenge of future technologies like these (along with all the others available to clinicians, banks, credit institutions, marketers, etc.) is how the comprehension and management of their data may precipitate safety threats, such as a health professional's wondering what a 38 percent probability of his patient's developing prostate cancer in the next ten years clinically entails. Bjørn Hofmann has noted how such technologically created knowledge will bring not only considerable benefit but considerable disutility.[4] On the positive side, as the sensitivity and specificity of diagnostic tests improve, more cases will be detected, testing will therefore increase, the number of persons diagnosed with a disease will also likely increase, and we may witness a revision in the understanding of the disease to include its milder forms, resulting in more diagnoses and more cases. Thus, the good news is that treatment outcomes will improve because of earlier detections, with more survivors and success stories, leading to increased use of the technologies.

But not all technologies nor their findings will boast such successes. Hofmann remarks that some technologies will be greeted with great enthusiasm before their efficacy is established or before their downsides are adequately appreciated. Increased testing will likely result in "incidentalomas" (or new and unexpected) findings, which may be extremely beneficial or may be utterly without clinical value and only cause patients worry. Of course, healthcare spending will skyrocket but oftentimes without any concomitant patient benefit, as diseases may be detected for which no treatments exist, or there may be overtreatment resulting in a net harm. Healthcare consumers might find all this perplexing, as some will benefit but many will not, causing worries among health experts on the undisciplined use of these technologies.

Consider, then, how such technologies affect vigilance, mindfulness, compliance, and humility. The vigilant health professional will keep a critical eye on interventions, treatment outcomes, and their risk-benefit ratios; mindfulness will require a keen self-scrutiny and evaluation of the reasons for recommending a treatment or not; compliance challenges will be legion as new technologies require new operational skills that may take considerable time to learn and may be resisted if the learning effort is arduous and without a personal payoff; and humility will persistently force the question of who is benefiting the most from such utilization: patients, clinicians, insurers, or drug and device manufacturers? Of course, relevant evaluative data may be inconclusive or incomplete while self-interest is bound to affect the evaluation process.

Until now, humans have coped with technological change relatively well or at least without allowing it to destroy ourselves. Unfortunately, though, since the Second World War, we have possessed the technology of global destruction, and presently, we can add to the specter of nuclear war the threat of climate change, cyberattacks that could eliminate resources on which large segments of human life depends (such as pulse bombs that disable everything using electricity), and biological warfare that could wipe out large segments of our populations. The world thus feels much less safe than previously, and we can only hope that our knowledge, wisdom, and good will can regulate and contain the large-scaled lethality of such technologies. Thus, this book's concern about safety in healthcare can be extrapolated to a global concern, while the book's reliance on its four structural constructs might suggest that vigilance be directed to global environmental threats; mindfulness to the assessment of the reasonableness of our beliefs and actions; compliance applied to international policies and practices that seek to realize a prosperous, peaceful, and ethical world; and humility directed especially toward reducing the hubris of world leaders and their supporters and accepting the wisdom and lessons of "bounded rationality."

As I prepare to enter my eighth decade, I'm struck by how life is a process of change. Virtually everything around and within us changes as we age: our families, friends, wealth, interests, abilities, aptitudes, health, the technologies we use, and our physical and spiritual environments. And then, of course, we begin the dying process and experience the last change of all.

What is particularly worrisome about the twenty-first century is that many of its technologies will be so innovative that we will have next to no idea as to their consequences or how to strategically manage their operations once they are unleashed and begin creating and delivering their products. Thus, we should expect increasingly shrill debates between risk-relishing futurists and risk-avoidant conservatives that may very well characterize the social and political conversation of Western cultures for decades to come. But ethics will look to us—since humans are the only life forms on the planet who can be ethically accountable—to shape our moralities in ethically defensible ways. One hopes that we will do so with a veneration for human reason, that is, with an unwavering insistence on beliefs, arguments, and reasonings that are logical, true to fact, and respectful of other intellectually earnest and informed points of view. Whether the topic is patient safety or the safety of the planet, to forsake reliable knowledge and reason, to understand human welfare as an individual rather than a collective pursuit, and to cede authority to others to shape our beliefs and actions would invite worldwide suffering, as history has abundantly taught. While democracy's greatest advantage is in enabling us to correct our mistakes through the political process, democracy also allows us to equip ourselves with the best available intelligence to avoid the kinds of mistakes that could require decades if not centuries to remedy.

Ultimately, the most valuable of the four constructs that anchor the chapters of this book may be humility. By acknowledging and understanding our imperfections, we are in a better position to compensate for them; we might be less inclined to hurt or harm when we are anxious or angry;

we might construct better networks of cooperation, trust, intelligence, and empathy; we might choose which sacrifices to make in a more informed and productive way; and we might more readily appreciate and advance an overall improvement in the quality of life on our planet. At the very least, we might all be safer.

Interview with Bob Wachter

Robert M. Wachter, MD, is a professor in and chair of the Department of Medicine at the University of California, San Francisco. He is the author or coauthor of 250 articles and 6 books. Wachter coined the term "hospitalist" in 1996 and is often considered the father of the hospitalist field, the fastest growing specialty in the history of modern medicine. He is past president of the Society of Hospital Medicine and past chair of the American Board of Internal Medicine. In the safety and quality arenas, he edits the US government's leading website on patient safety and has written two books on the subject, *Internal Bleeding* and *Understanding Patient Safety*, the world's best-selling safety primer. In 2004, he received the John M. Eisenberg Award, the nation's top honor in patient safety. In 2015, *Modern Healthcare* magazine ranked him as the most influential physician-executive in the United States. He has served on the healthcare advisory boards of several companies, including Google. His 2015 book, *The Digital Doctor: Hope, Hype and Harm at the Dawn of Medicine's Computer Age*, was a *New York Times* science best seller. He recently chaired a blue ribbon commission advising England's National Health Service on its digital strategy.

JB: Bob, thanks so much for taking the time to do this interview. The first and maybe most pressing question I have for you is this: Throughout this book, I'm wanting to make a case for cultivating foreseeability, or what James Reason has called "feral vigilance." So I'm promoting the need for health professionals to develop a hazard awareness or error wisdom about their environments and their own thinking. Yet, I'm seriously wondering whether this is a plausible or realistic proposal. I hear a lot of health professionals saying they are just too busy to be thoughtful to that kind of degree. Others say that you first need a brush with hazard to appreciate where it lies; you can't predict or prognosticate it. So, on this continuum of pessimism to optimism about cultivating hazard awareness, what do you believe is possible?

RW: Like most complex questions, I think the answer is somewhere in between. There are a lot of risks that are unforeseeable, and they sometimes relate to the most benign of conditions. When you go back, it may or may not have been obvious that there were risky conditions, but often it wasn't obvious until the error happened. Afterward, people would look and say, "The way the computer screen was organized was risky." But to characterize all risks that way—that we always identify them in hindsight—would mean that everything is risky . . . and therefore nothing is risky. And yet, I think a lot about patient safety, so I may be more sensitive to these things than others. But I'm pretty confident that people can be taught to have a mindset about latent and risky conditions so that when they see them—like a case where there are a lot of doctors involved, or we're using an unusual medicine, or the patient is tenuous and has to go down to the radiology department, or when a laboratory report comes back and is really, really weird—in the old days, I don't know that I'd have said, "Could that be wrong?" But for many people today, it's become instinctive to scan the environment and do what you can to prophylax for hazards. I think it can be taught to some extent, although to some extent it truly is experience—you've seen screw-ups, so you know that certain situations can be risky. But I think there are a lot of errors—probably the majority—that just came out of the blue; nobody reasonable could have anticipated their causes, and you have to figure out how to learn from them so as to error-proof the situation for the next person.

JB: So, it seems reasonable to think that in so many situations, the hazards are not foreseeable, but once a clinician has learned that there is this hazard or error trap in the environment, that experience may sensitize you to that environment so that you'll be more cautious.

RW: Also, I think you have to separate out individual learning from organizational learning. One of the key challenges for an organization is how to increase the probability that an individual will see an unsafe condition and act rather than take the easier way, which is to say, "Oh, that's not safe. I'll just be more careful next time." Of course, it takes time and energy to report it to someone and have the confidence that that will be a meaningful act. So, there are two ways for individuals to respond to unsafe conditions: that there is an organizational mechanism that will result in organizational learning and improvement through reporting, and there's the more individual one, with people saying, "Oh, that's a risky situation that predisposes to an error," which then triggers individual vigilance but it doesn't result in organizational change. So, yes, you do want people to be vigilant and recognize unsafe conditions, but then there's the next consideration, which is what do they do—

make a personal change or go the extra step and seek some organizational action about it?

JB: That's a great point. I want to add a third consideration or problem, though: I'm very taken with the production pressures that our health professionals are under. A clinician said to me about a month ago that "sometimes it feels like we're workers on an assembly line at an automobile plant. We just go through the motions without thinking, because if you would stop to think, you'd fall behind." So, the production pressures just serve to blunt your hazard awareness and sensitivities. What do you think about that?

RW: No question that people today are running pretty fast, probably faster than they used to. I think the stresses on humans have increased as the electronic data systems require additional inputs and pathways, which you can then access all the time. So, when you feel those pressures, many people will put blinders on to get to the next task. The problem, of course, is that those kinds of production pressures will make organizational reporting of safety hazards less likely. In fact, reporting or calling organizational attention to them becomes an act of altruism because it's relatively unlikely that you will encounter such a risk in your own patient care. So you do it for the sake of others. But acts of altruism tend not to occur when you're very busy. Also, you can say to yourself that it's very unlikely that the hazard you spot is going to kill somebody tomorrow. And even if someone is harmed, it's probably not going to be one of your patients, or it's probably not going to be on your watch, or you're never going to hear about it. So, the calculus of "Do I take two minutes to report that situation given the low probability that the benefit will accrue to my patient?" is going to drop the chance of you reporting the error or condition down pretty close to zero.

Actually, I don't think that even with tight blinders on, clinicians will miss these potential hazards. They will register them. But what I do think is more likely is burnout. You're really, really busy; you're feeling fried; you're just trying to get through. That sort of pressure probably harms the learning quality of the institution more than it harms the individual's ability to perceive and register a hazardous condition.

JB: OK. Let me just throw some topics at you and get your reactions. You mentioned health information technologies, and I happen to have a copy of a *Health Affairs* article that you wrote and that came out in 2010, "Patient Safety at Ten: Unmistakable Progress, Troubling Gaps." So, here we are seven years later, and I'm interested in your take on health information technologies. I can tell you that wherever I go, when the talk turns to electronic health records, I hear nothing good. Nothing.

RW: Originally, we thought the computer was going to make our lives much better, but it seems that all we got from a provider's standpoint was having to spend more time inputting data and not getting much out. So, two years ago I wrote *The Digital Doctor*, frankly out of frustration because I initially shared the utopian hope that computers would make our work easier and better and safer. And I was frankly shocked to see how unhappy these technologies were making people. We had a terrible error occur some years ago at UCSF involving a drug overdose. It happened in a fully electronic system, where the technology was doing what it was supposed to do, and the clinicians were doing what they were supposed to do. The machine's alerts were firing away but were being ignored because they do that thousands of times a day, and it never seems to amount to anything. So there was this slow motion train wreck happening right in front of everyone. And it became clear to me that computers can solve certain problems, but they also can make new ones. At the end of my book, I discuss a concept called the "Productivity Paradox of IT," which basically says that the first 5 to 10 years of digitization in a given industry tends not to yield the benefits that people expect. But then, somewhere around year 10 (although in healthcare it may be year 15 because we're more complicated), you start seeing the benefits. The reason that it takes that long is because nobody is smart enough to do anything with the technology except to re-create the work they used to do in analog. But as they become more familiar with the technology over time, they begin thinking about the nature of the work and the nature of the task in different ways and become less tethered to the old ways of doing things. They get more creative and ambitious about reimagining the whole process using digital tools. That's when you start seeing massive gains. So my feeling is that we're about 5 years into the widespread digitization of healthcare, and while it has created more new work, it has solved more errors than it's created. Still, the systems are clunky. But I'm starting to see things getting better. Like so many other institutions, we bought the Epic system, which is basically a big data repository machine. It doesn't do many of the things you'd want a computer system to do, like help you make diagnoses, help you review thousands of patients in the chart to get you what you need, and alert you in a way that doesn't overalert you. Now, I don't think it's Epic's job to solve all these things, as they did a reasonably good job building the best-selling EHR [electronic health record]. But now Silicon Valley is getting interested in all this. These digital companies and start-ups are realizing that clinical care may begin with the EHR, but then the solutions need to come from other products that complement the EHR. But once those technologies do start appearing, I think we're going to see diagnostic artificial intelligence, better predictions, better use of voice recognition, much more sophisticated searches of the EHR, and better integration with the clinical literature. All of that seems to me inevitable.

JB: And now we're seeing neural network recognition technologies where people like Sebastian Thrun are training algorithms to categorize skin lesions with an accuracy that is just as good if not better than board-certified dermatologists.

RW: There's no question in my mind that the current model of an expert looking at a visual pattern, say, in radiology or dermatology, and saying that looks like X will be challenged by technology in the next 5 years and probably completely overtaken by the technology in the next 10 to 15 years. But you need to realize that's different from a patient coming into my office and my making a better diagnosis. The idea of looking at a bunch of dots on an x-ray, or a skin lesion, or a pathology assessment is in AI's sweet spot. But for Watson to win on *Jeopardy*, the computer had to solve a riddle after being given 2 to 4 items. Contrast that with a patient coming into the ER with pain, at which point the doctor will elicit and need to consider perhaps 200 data points. The act of distilling these 200 down to the 4 or 5 salient ones that I'm going to act on turns out to be really hard. What's likely going to happen is the human operator will choose 4 or 5 variables that he thinks are the salient ones and then ask the computer, "Well, computer, what do you think?" And I think computers will respond reasonably well. What they'll do is decrease diagnostic errors by prompting you to think about something you've not considered. It's one thing to perform pattern recognition; it's quite another to do clinical diagnosis, which is much harder.

JB: So, you mentioned in your 2010 *Health Affairs* article that you were disappointed with physician involvement in patient safety. What are your thoughts now? Are you seeing physicians embracing the strategies of patient safety, or are you still seeing a lack of involvement?

RW: It may be worse now. The physician burnout issue is very real. Now 17 years into the patient safety movement, you can't say to people any more,

"If you really work hard, there will be a payoff in the end not only for patient safety but for your own work satisfaction. It will have a personal benefit for you." We just haven't seen that. And I'm worried about patient safety
in another way: When the patient safety movement began, it was the only
quality-improvement game in town. Suppose you were a physician who happened to be interested in improvement and didn't mind taking time off from
clinical work to go to meetings, to learn about the initiatives, to champion
their implementation, and so forth. Today that same physician is much bus-
ier and is no longer being measured on just safety but on a host of quality
variables and measures. There's also efficiency and "Choosing Wisely" [i.e.,
reducing waste] and cost reduction and patient satisfaction. So, even if you
were among that fairly small group of physicians who are interested in quality
and participating on committees that focus on that, you're being pulled in a
lot of directions today. So, I see trainees coming in who are more interested
in safety and quality than their predecessors, but they are also going to be
asked, "Are you a person who wants to work on process improvement, using
a method like Lean? Are you an IT person? Are you a patient experience person? A quality person?" So safety work is going to be competing against these
other improvement imperatives. While that might be a good thing in a way,
this competition will reduce efforts to improve safety. On the other hand, it
might be the case that the more general quality-improvement efforts we do
will lower errors and improve safety as a collateral benefit. But the number of
people who primarily want to do safety as their primary focus is less than it
was 5 or 10 years ago.

JB: So, let's end on an optimistic note: What are you excited about, optimistic
about, enthusiastic about as you look toward the next 5 to 10 years on patient
safety and the quality-improvement things you were talking about?

RW: Well, I think our prospects for improving our healthcare systems in the
near future are greater than they were when the patient safety movement
got started. All these safety and quality initiatives involving the payment environment, the accreditation environment, the transparency environment,
the satisfaction environment—which are tied with money to support these
efforts—have sensitized us to decreasing readmissions, committing fewer errors, having patients more satisfied, or reducing infections. So, these pressures have created momentum for improvement across all the dimensions
of value. And that's been good. Moreover, we've professionalized a lot of the
work. At a place like UCSF, we have a chief quality officer, chief patient safety

officer, chief patient experience officer, and these people have built levels of institutional competency and infrastructures that we haven't had before.

But the biggest hope for me is in informatics. A lot of errors that we have seen have involved information not moving around seamlessly, or getting dropped, or people not having information when they need it. I've come to learn that the disappointment of the first 5 years of IT is not that surprising. In fact, it's sort of what improvement looks like. In the beginning the tools will be clunky, people will put them in without much thought about workflow, user interfaces, and culture. So, I think we're getting to the end of "Why, that's surprising; I didn't expect that" and beginning a phase where we're going to see more innovative tools being used in a more thoughtful way, driven in part by a healthcare system where the pressures are constantly on delivering better value. So, I think this is going to take another 5 to 10 years, but at the end of it, we're going to see a lot of improvement promoted by more effective use of IT, on top of all of the other individual and organizational competencies and cultural changes.

JB: Bob, thank you so much. This was great.

RW: You're welcome.

References

Preface

1. Beauchamp TL, Childress JF. *Principles of Biomedical Ethics*. 7th ed. New York: Oxford University Press; 2013.

2. Hollnagel E, Wears RL, Braithwaite J. 2015. *From Safety-I to Safety-II: A White Paper*. Odense: Resilient Health Care Net, University of Southern Denmark; Jacksonville: University of Florida; and Sydney: Macquarie University; 2015. https://www.england.nhs.uk/signuptosafety/wp-content/uploads/sites/16/2015/10/safety-1-safety-2-whte-papr.pdf.

3. Cook R; Cognitive Technologies Laboratory, University of Chicago. How complex systems fail. http://web.mit.edu/2.75/resources/random/How%20Complex%20Systems%20Fail.pdf. Updated as Revision D (00.04.21) in 2000.

Chapter 1. Ethical Foundations of Patient Safety

1. Reason J. *Human Error*. Cambridge: Cambridge University Press; 1990.

2. Beauchamp TL, Childress JF. *Principles of Biomedical Ethics*. 7th ed. New York: Oxford University Press; 2013.

3. Smith CM. Origin and uses of *primum non nocere*—Above all, do no harm! *Journal of Clinical Pharmacology*. 2005;45:371-77.

4. Pierce EC. Looking back: Doctor Pierce reflects (An excerpt from the 1995 Emery A. Rovenstine Lecture). *APSF Newsletter*. 2007;22(1). http://www.apsf.org/newsletters/html/2007/spring/02_looking_back.htm.

5. Lanier WL. A three-decade perspective on anesthesia safety. *American Surgeon*. 2006;72(11):985-89.

6. Kohn LT, Corrigan JM, Donaldson MS. *To Err Is Human: Building a Safer Health System*. Washington, DC: National Academy Press; 1999.

7. Brennan TA, Leape LL, Laird NM, et al. Incidence of adverse events and negligence in hospitalized patients: Results of the Harvard Medical Practice Study I. *New England Journal of Medicine*. 1991;324:370-76.

8. Leape LL. Scope of problem and history of patient safety. *Obstetrics and Gynecology Clinics of North America*. 2008;35:1-10.

9. Weinstein MM. Checking medicine's vital signs. *New York Times Magazine*. April 19, 1998. http://www.nytimes.com/1998/04/19/magazine/checking-medicine-s-vital-signs.html.

10. Meyer GS, Battles J, Hart JC, Tang N. The US Agency for Healthcare Research and Quality's activities in patient safety research. *International Journal for Quality in Healthcare*. 2003;15(1):i25-i30.

11. Banja J. *Medical Errors and Medical Narcissism*. Sudbury, MA: Jones and Bartlett; 2005.

12. Banja J. Does medical error disclosure violate the medical malpractice insurance cooperation clause? In Henriksen K, Battles JB, Marks E, Lewin DI, eds. *Advances in Patient Safety: From Research to Implementation.* Rockville, MD: Agency for Healthcare Research and Quality and Department of Defense—Health Affairs; 2005:371–81. AHRQ Publication No. 05-0021-3. http://www.ahrq.gov/sites/default /files/wysiwyg/professionals/quality-patient-safety/patient-safety-resources /resources/advances-in-patient-safety/vol3/Banja.pdf.

13. Boothman R, Blackwell A, Campbell D, et al. A better approach to medical malpractice claims? The University of Michigan experience. *Journal of Health and Life Sciences Law.* 2009;2:125–59.

14. Benn J, Koutantji M, Wallace L, et al. Feedback from incident reporting: Information and action to improve patient safety. *Quality and Safety in Healthcare.* 2009;18:11–21.

15. MacIntyre A. *After Virtue.* Notre Dame, IN: University of Notre Dame Press; 1981.

16. Bayles MD. *Professional Ethics.* 2nd ed. Belmont, CA: Wadsworth; 1989.

17. Reeves AR. Standard threats: How to violate basic human rights. *Social Theory and Practice.* 2015;41(3):403–34.

18. Kant I. *Groundwork of the Metaphysic of Morals.* Paton HJ, trans. New York: Harper Torchbooks; 1964.

19. Walker R. *Kant.* New York: Routledge; 1999.

20. Aronfeld SM. Sexual assault by a healthcare provider. *Trial.* Dec. 2009:46–50.

21. Tavris C, Aronson E. *Mistakes Were Made (But Not by Me).* Orlando, FL: Harcourt; 2007.

22. Waterman AD, Garbutt J, Hazel E, et al. The emotional impact of medical errors on practicing physicians in the United States and Canada. *Joint Commission Journal on Quality and Patient Safety.* 2007;33(8):467–76.

23. Shortell SM, Singer SJ. Improving patient safety by taking systems seriously. *JAMA.* 2008;299(4):445–47.

24. Owen DG. Figuring foreseeability. *Wake Forest Law Review.* 2009;44:1277–1307.

25. Mullin R. Cost to develop new pharmaceutical drugs now exceeds $2.5B. *Scientific American.* Nov. 24, 2014. https://www.scientificamerican.com/article/cost -to-develop-new-pharmaceutical-drug-now-exceeds-2-5b/.

26. Reason J. *The Human Contribution.* Burlington, VT: Ashgate; 2008.

27. Sinnott-Armstrong W. Consequentialism. *Stanford Encyclopedia of Philosophy.* http://plato.stanford.edu/entries/consequentialism/. Revised Oct. 22, 2015.

28. Cohen E, Bonifield J. Secret deaths: CNN finds high surgical death rate for children at a Florida hospital. CNN.com. http://www.cnn.com/2015/06/01/health /st-marys-medical-center/. Published June 15, 2015.

29. Cohen E, Bonifield J. CNN report on high mortality rate for babies at Florida hospital leads to inquiry. CNN.com. http://www.cnn.com/2015/06/05/health /st-marys-medical-center-investigation/. Published June 8, 2015.

30. Cohen E. CNN report on Florida hospital leads to heart surgery program

closure. CNN.com. http://www.cnn.com/2015/08/17/health/st-marys-medical
-center-investigation/. Published Aug. 19, 2015.

31. Cohen E, Bonifield J. What to know about St. Mary's children's heart
surgery mortality rates. CNN.com. http://www.cnn.com/2015/06/09/health
/childrens-heart-surgery-mortality-rates-qa/. Published July 1, 2015.

32. Wemple E. CNN faces lawsuit over exposé on Florida hospital. *Washington Post.* Feb. 16, 2016. https://www.washingtonpost.com/blogs/erik-wemple
/wp/2016/02/16/cnn-faces-lawsuit-over-expose-on-florida-hospital/?utm_term
=.a5b7573612cc.

33. Aristotle. *Nicomachean Ethics.* In Jenkinson AJ, trans.; McKeon R, ed. *The Basic Works of Aristotle.* New York: Random House; 1970:935-1112.

34. Triandis H. *Fooling Ourselves.* Westport, CT: Praeger; 2009.

35. Institute for Safe Medication Practices. Side tracks on the safety express:
Interruptions leading to errors and unfinished . . . Wait, what was I doing?" *Acute Care ISMP Medication Safety Alert.* Nov. 29, 2012. https://www.ismp.org/resources
/side-tracks-safety-express-interruptions-lead-errors-and-unfinished-wait-what
-was-i-doing.

Chapter 2. Vigilance

1. Hollnagel E, Wears RL, Braithwaite J. *From Safety-I to Safety-II: A White Paper.*
Odense: Resilient Health Care Net, University of Southern Denmark; Jacksonville: University of Florida; and Sydney: Macquarie University; 2015. https://www
.england.nhs.uk/signuptosafety/wp-content/uploads/sites/16/2015/10/safety-1-safety
-2-whte-papr.pdf.

2. Gabbard G. The role of compulsiveness in the normal physician. *JAMA.*
1985;254(20):2926-29.

3. Oxford University Press. Vigilant (adj.). *Oxford Living Dictionaries.* https://
en.oxforddictionaries.com/definition/vigilant. Accessed Oct. 6, 2018.

4. Comarow A. Jesica's story. *US News and World Report.* July 28-Aug. 4,
2003;135(3):51-73.

5. Altman LK. Big doses of chemotherapy drug killed patient, hurt 2d. *New York Times.* March 24, 1995. http://www.nytimes.com/1995/03/24/us/big-doses
-of-chemotherapy-drug-killed-patient-hurt-2d.html.

6. Reason J. *The Human Contribution.* Burlington, VT: Ashgate; 2008.

7. WhiteCoatDO. Like drinking water from a fire hose. *WhiteCoatDO.* http://
www.whitecoatdo.com/like-drinking-water-from-a-fire-hose/. Published Aug. 27,
2012.

8. Owen DG. Figuring foreseeability. *Wake Forest Law Review.* 2009;44:1277-1307.

9. Banja JD. Failures of foreseeability: Risk management considerations in reducing allegations of sexual violence in psychiatric units. *Journal of Health Care Risk Management.* 2016;36(3):21-25.

10. Cook R; Cognitive Technologies Laboratory, University of Chicago. How
complex systems fail. http://web.mit.edu/2.75/resources/random/How%20Complex%20Systems%20Fail.pdf. Updated as Revision D (00.04.21) in 2000.

11. LeDoux J. *The Emotional Brain.* New York: Simon and Schuster; 1998.

12. Reason J. *The Human Contribution.* Burlington, VT: Ashgate; 2008.

13. Simon HA, Egidi M, Marris RL, Viale R. *Economics, Bounded Rationality and the Cognitive Revolution.* Brookfield, VT: Elgar; 1992.

14. Beauchamp TL, Childress JF. *Principles of Biomedical Ethics.* 7th ed. New York: Oxford University Press; 2013.

15. Feinberg J. *Harm to Others: The Moral Limits of the Criminal Law.* New York: Oxford University Press; 1984.

16. Pronovost PJ, Goeschel CA, Wachter RM. The wisdom and justice of not paying for "preventable complications." *JAMA.* 2008;299(18):2197-99.

17. Banja J. When harms become wrongs: Some comments on the moral language of oppression and the limitations of moral theory. *Journal of Disability Policy Studies.* 2001;12(2):79-86.

18. Powers M, Faden R. *Social Justice: The Moral Foundations of Public Health and Health Policy.* New York: Oxford University Press; 2006.

19. Harbin T. *Waking Up Blind: Lawsuits over Eye Surgery.* Minneapolis, MN: Langdon Street Press; 2009.

20. Golding D, Tuler S. Risk and risk assessment. In Jennings B, ed. *Encyclopedia of Bioethics.* 4th ed. Farmington Mills, MI: Macmillan Reference; 2014:2873-81.

21. Vrilling JK, van Hengel W, Houben RJ. Acceptable risk as a basis for design. *Reliability Engineering and System Safety.* 1998;59:141-50.

22. Jonsen AR, Siegler M, Winslade WJ. *Clinical Ethics.* 7th ed. New York: McGraw-Hill Medical; 2010:51-60.

23. Phelps AC, Maciejewski PK, Nilsson M, et al. Religious coping and use of intensive life-prolonging care near death in patients with advanced cancer. *JAMA.* 2009;301(11):1140-47.

24. Periyakoil VS, Neri E, Fong A, Kraemer H. Do unto others: Doctors' personal end-of-life resuscitation preferences and their attitudes toward advance directives. PLoS ONE 2014;9(5):e98246. http://journals.plos.org/plosone/article?id=10.1371/journal.pone.0098246.

25. Cook R, Rasmussen J. "Going solid": A model for system dynamics and consequences for patient safety. *Quality and Safety in Health Care.* April 5, 2005:130-34.

26. Gerstein M. *Flirting with Disaster: Why Accidents Are Rarely Accidental.* New York: Union Square Press; 2008.

27. Pronovost PJ, Colantuoni E. Measuring preventable harm: Helping science keep pace with policy. *JAMA.* 2009;301(12):1273-75.

28. Bal BS. An introduction to medical malpractice in the United States. *Clinical Orthopedics and Related Research.* 2009;467(2):339-47.

29. Xu T. Mortality risks associated with emergency admission during weekends and public holidays. *Hospitalist.* https://www.the-hospitalist.org/hospitalist/article/151089/transitions-care/mortality-risks-associated-emergency-admission-during. Published Nov. 3, 2017.

30. Reason J. *Human Error.* Cambridge: Cambridge University Press; 1990.

31. Howe P. *Leadership and Training for the Fight*. Bloomington, IN: Author House; 2005.

32. Henneman EA, Gawlinski A, Blank FS, et al. Strategies used by critical care nurses to identify, interrupt, and correct medical errors. *American Journal of Critical Care*. 2010;19(6):500–509.

33. National Academies of Sciences, Engineering, and Medicine; Institute of Medicine. *Improving Diagnosis in Health Care*. Balogh EP, Miller BT, Ball J, eds. Washington, DC: National Academies Press; 2015. https://www.nap.edu/catalog /21794/improving-diagnosis-in-health-care.

34. Nouri SS, Rudd RE. Health literacy in the "oral exchange": An important element of patient-provider communication. *Patient Education and Counseling*. 2015;98(5):565–71.

35. Robert Wood Johnson Foundation. OpenNotes. https://www.rwjf.org/en /how-we-work/grants-explorer/featured-programs/opennotes.html. Accessed Oct. 6, 2018.

36. H. G. Wells. Quotes. Quotable Quote. Goodreads.com. http://www.good reads.com/quotes/107797-civilization-is-in-a-race-between-education-and-catastro phe-let. Accessed Oct. 6, 2018.

37. Cook RI, Nemeth CP. "Those found responsible have been sacked": Some observations on the usefulness of error. *Cognition, Technology and Work*. 2010;12(2): 87–93.

38. Boodman SG. Diagnosing medical errors: In the wake of widely publi-cized mistakes, doctors try to make hospitals safer. *Washington Post*. Nov. 19, 1996. https://www.washingtonpost.com/archive/lifestyle/wellness/1996/11/19/diagnosing -medical-errors-in-the-wake-of-widely-publicized-mistakes-doctors-try-to-make -hospitals-safer/089db0e9-c65b-4cd9-b345-02f332a5c011/?utm_term=.95e462bb1fd3.

39. Cook RI, Woods DD, Miller CA. *A Tale of Two Stories: Contrasting Views of Patient Safety*. Report from a workshop on Assembling the Scientific Basis for Progress on Patient Safety; National Health Care Safety Council of the NPSF at the AMA; Jan. 1998. https://www.researchgate.net/publication/245102691_A_Tale_of _Two_Stories_Contrasting_Views_of_Patient_Safety.

Chapter 3. Mindfulness

1. Croskerry P. Bias: A normal operating characteristic of the diagnosing brain. *Diagnosis*. 2014;1(1):23–27.

2. Lommel K. Twitter, April 4, 2016, 8:40 a.m. https://twitter.com/karenlommel /status/716983795623309312.

3. Rich BA. Medical custom and medical ethics: Rethinking the standard of care. *Cambridge Quarterly of Healthcare Ethics*. 2005;14:27–39.

4. Mehlman MJ. Professional power and the standard of care in medicine. *Ari-zona State Law Journal*. 2012;44:1165–1235.

5. Harari Y. *Homo Deus*. New York: HarperCollins; 2017:308–402.

6. Allain J. From *Jeopardy!* to jaundice: The medical liability implications

of Dr. Watson and other artificial intelligence systems. *Louisiana Law Review.* 2013;73(4):1049-79.

7. Graber M, Kissam S, Payne VL, et al. Cognitive interventions to reduce diagnostic error: A narrative review. *BMJ Quality and Safety.* 2012;21(7):535-57.

8. Teper R, Segal ZV, Inzlicht M. Inside the mindful mind: How mindfulness enhances emotion regulation through improvements in executive control. *Current Directions in Psychological Science.* 2013;22(6):449-54.

9. National Academies of Sciences, Engineering, and Medicine; Institute of Medicine. *Improving Diagnosis in Health Care.* Balogh EP, Miller BT, Ball J, eds. Washington, DC: National Academies Press; 2015. https://www.nap.edu/catalog /21794/improving-diagnosis-in-health-care.

10. Hoffman J; CRICO Strategies. *2014 Annual Benchmarking Report: Malpractice Risks in the Diagnostic Process.* Cambridge, MA: CRICO Strategies; 2014. https:// psnet.ahrq.gov/resources/resource/28612/2014-annual-benchmarking-report-mal practice-risks-in-the-diagnostic-process.

11. Berner ES, Graber ML. Overconfidence as a cause of diagnostic error in medicine. *American Journal of Medicine.* 2008;121(5A):S2-S23.

12. Mamede S, van Gog T, van der Berge K, et al. Effect of availability bias and reflective reasoning on diagnostic accuracy among internal medicine residents. *JAMA.* 2010;304(11):1198-1203.

13. Singh H, Giardina TD, Meyer A, et al. Types and origins of diagnostic errors in primary care settings. *JAMA Internal Medicine.* 2013;173(6):418-23.

14. Graber ML, Franklin N, Gordon R. Diagnostic error in internal medicine. *Archives of Internal Medicine.* 2005;165(13):1493-99.

15. Miles RW. Fallacious reasoning and complexity as root causes of clinical inertia. *Journal of the American Medical Directors Association.* 2007;8(6):349-54.

16. Levinson W, Kao A, Kuby A, Thisted RA. Not all patients want to participate in decision making. *Journal of General Internal Medicine.* 2005;20(6):531-35.

17. Delbanco T, Bell SK. Guilty, afraid, and alone—Struggling with medical error. *New England Journal of Medicine.* 2007;357(17):1682-83.

18. Reason J. *The Human Contribution.* Burlington, VT: Ashgate; 2008.

19. Schiff GD, Hasan O, Kim S, et al. Diagnostic error in medicine. *Archives of Internal Medicine.* 2009;169(20):1881-87.

20. Mankad K, Hoey ETD, Jones JB, Tirukonda P, Smith JT. Radiology errors: Are we learning from our mistakes? *Clinical Radiology.* 2009;64:988-993.

21. Wears RL, Nemeth CP. Replacing hindsight with insight: Toward better understanding of diagnostic failure. *Annals of Emergency Medicine.* 2007;49(2):206-9.

22. Lockley SW, Barger LK, Ayas NT, et al. Effects of health care provider work hours and sleep deprivation on safety and performance. *Joint Commission Journal on Quality and Patient Safety.* 2007;33(11)(suppl):7-18. http://media.npr.org/assets /news/2016/04/sleep.pdf.

23. Kahneman D. *Thinking Fast and Slow.* New York: Farrar, Straus and Giroux; 2011.

24. Triandis H. *Fooling Ourselves.* Westport, CT: Praeger; 2009.

25. Gandhi TK, Kachalia A, Thomas EJ, et al. Missed and delayed diagnoses

in the ambulatory setting: A study of closed malpractice claims. *Annals of Internal Medicine.* 2006;145(7):488-96.

26. Croskerry P. Cognitive forcing strategies in clinical decision making. *Annals of Emergency Medicine.* 2003;41(1):110-20.

27. Simon HA, Egidi M, Marris RL, Viale R. *Economics, Bounded Rationality and the Cognitive Revolution.* Brookfield, VT: Elgar; 1992.

28. Johnson DDP, Blumstein DT, Fowler JH, Haselton MG. The evolution of error: Error management, cognitive constrains, and adaptive decision-making biases. *Trends in Ecology and Evolution.* 2013;28(8):474-81.

29. Jena A, Schoemaker L, Bhattacharya J, Seabury S. Physician spending and subsequent risk of malpractice claims: Observational study. *BMJ.* 2015;351:h5516.

30. Banja J. *Medical Errors and Medical Narcissism.* Sudbury, MA: Jones and Bartlett; 2005.

31. Owens BP, Johnson MD, Mitchell TR. Expressed humility in organizations: Implications for performance, teams, and leadership. *Organization Science.* 2013;24(5):1517-38.

32. Novack D, Suchman AL, Clark W, Epstein RM, Najberg E, Kaplan C. Calibrating the physician: Personal awareness and effective patient care. *JAMA.* 1997;278(8):502-9.

33. Lipson M, Lipson A. Psychotherapy and the ethics of attention. *Hastings Center Report.* 1996;26(1):17-22.

34. ECRI Institute and ISMP. Diagnostic error in acute care. *Pennsylvania Patient Safety Advisory.* 2010;7(3):76-86. http://patientsafety.pa.gov/ADVISORIES/Pages/201009_76.aspx.

35. Croskerry P. From mindfulness to mindful practice—cognitive bias and clinical decision making. *New England Journal of Medicine.* 2013;368(26):2445-48.

36. Levy N. Rethinking neuroethics in the light of the extended mind thesis. *American Journal of Bioethics.* 2007;7(9):3-11.

37. Ridderikhoff J, van Herk B. Who is afraid of the system? Doctors' attitude towards diagnostic systems. *International Journal of Medical Informatics.* 1998;53(1999):91-100.

38. Bostrom N. *Superintelligence: Paths, Dangers, Strategies.* Oxford: Oxford University Press; 2014.

39. Allyn J, Gabarro R, Roy P, et al. 2011. *Sentinel Events: Annual Report to the Joint Standing Committee on Health and Human Services, Maine State Legislature.* Augusta, ME: Division of Licensing and Regulatory Services, 2011. https://www1.maine.gov/dhhs/reports/sentinel_events_report.pdf.

40. El-Kareh R, Hasan O, Schiff GD. 2013. Use of health information technology to reduce diagnostic errors [published online ahead of print Aug. 7, 2013]. *BMJ Quality and Safety.* http://qualitysafety.bmj.com/content/early/2013/08/07/bmjqs-2013-001884.

41. Cook R; Cognitive Technologies Laboratory, University of Chicago. How complex systems fail. http://web.mit.edu/2.75/resources/random/How%20Complex%20Systems%20Fail.pdf. Updated as Revision D (00.04.21) in 2000.

42. Vladek DC. Machines without principals: Liability rules and artificial intelligence. *Washington Law Review.* 2014;89:117-50.

43. Ende J. Feedback in clinical medical education. *JAMA.* 1983;250(6):777-81.

44. Schiff GD. Minimizing diagnostic error: The importance of follow-up and feedback. *American Journal of Medicine.* 2008;121(5)(suppl):S38-S42.

45. Rudolph JW, Morrison JB. Sidestepping superstitious learning, ambiguity, and other roadblocks: A feedback model of diagnostic problem solving. *American Journal of Medicine.* 2008;121(5A):S34-S37.

46. Anderson PAM. Giving feedback on clinical skills: Are we starving our young? *Journal of Graduate Medical Education.* June 2012:154-58.

47. Gigante J, Dell M, Sharkey A. Getting beyond "good job": How to give effective feedback. *Pediatrics.* 2011;127:205-7.

48. Cantillon P, Sargeant J. Giving feedback in clinical settings. *BMJ.* 2008;337: 1292-94.

49. Brinko KT. The practice of giving feedback to improve teaching: What is effective? *Journal of Higher Education.* 1993;64(5):574-93.

50. Ramani S, Krackov SK. Twelve tips for giving feedback effectively in the clinical environment. *Medical Teacher.* 2012;34:787-91.

51. Shojania K, Burton EC, McDonald KM, Goldman L. Changes in rates of autopsy-detected diagnostic errors over time: A systematic review. *JAMA.* 2003;289(21):2849-56.

52. Chassin MR, Becher EC. The wrong patient. *Annals of Internal Medicine.* 2002;136:826-33.

53. Gawande A. Personal best: Top athletes and singers have coaches. Should you? *New Yorker.* Oct. 3, 2011. http://www.newyorker.com/magazine/2011/10/03 /personal-best.

54. Epstein R. Mindful practice. *JAMA.* 1999;282(9):833-39.

55. Sibinga EMS, Wu AW. Clinician mindfulness and patient safety. *JAMA.* 2010;304(22):2532-33.

Chapter 4. Compliance

Acknowledgment: This chapter originally appeared in the Elsevier journal *Business Horizons* in 2010 (volume 53, pages 139-48). Elsevier graciously permitted its being reprinted in this volume. Supported in part by PHS Grant UL1 RR025008 from the Clinical and Translational Science Award Program, National Institutes of Health, National Center for Research Resources.

1. Cook R; Cognitive Technologies Laboratory, University of Chicago. How complex systems fail. http://web.mit.edu/2.75/resources/random/How%20Com plex%20Systems%20Fail.pdf. Updated as Revision D (00.04.21) in 2000.

2. Gerstein M. *Flirting with Disaster: Why Accidents Are Rarely Accidental.* New York: Union Square Press; 2008.

3. Green M. Nursing error and human nature. *Journal of Nursing Law.* 2004;9(4):37-44.

4. Perrow C. *Normal Accidents: Living with High-Risk Technologies.* Princeton, NJ: Princeton University Press; 1999.

5. Reason J. *Human Error*. Cambridge: Cambridge University Press; 1990.

6. Woolf SH, Kuzel AJ, Dovey SM, Phillips RL. A string of mistakes: The importance of cascade analysis in describing, counting, and preventing medical errors. *Annals of Family Medicine*. 2004;2(4):317-26.

7. Vaughan DS. Organizational rituals of risk and error. In Hunter B and Power M, eds., *Organizational Encounters with Risk*. New York: Cambridge University Press; 2004:33-66.

8. Vaughan DS, Gleave EP, Welser HT. Controlling the evolution of corruption: Emulation, sanction, and prestige. Paper presented at the American Sociological Association Annual Meeting; Aug. 12, 2005; Philadelphia, PA. http://citation.allac ademic.com/meta/p_mla_apa_research_citation/0/2/2/8/2/pages22829/p22829-1 .php.

9. Maxfield D, Grenny J, Patterson K, McMillan R, Switzler A. Dialogue heals: The seven crucial conversations for the healthcare professional [discussion topics and recommendations based on the study *Silence Kills*]. Provo, UT: VitalSmarts; 2005. http://faculty.medicine.umich.edu/sites/default/files/resources/dialogue _heals.pdf.

10. Chassin MR, Becher EC. The wrong patient. *Annals of Internal Medicine*. 2002;136:826-33.

11. Banja J. *Medical Errors and Medical Narcissism*. Sudbury, MA: Jones and Bartlett; 2005.

12. Predmore S. The normalization of deviance. Keynote address at the of the American Association of Airport Executives Annual Meeting; Aug. 22, 2006; St. Louis, MO.

13. Vaughan DS. The dark side of organizations: Mistakes, misconduct, and disaster. *Annual Review of Sociology*. 1999;25:271-305.

14. Ashforth DE, Anand V. The normalization of corruption in organizations. *Research in Organizational Behavior*. 2003;25:1-52.

15. Kelly B. Preserving moral integrity: A follow-up study with new graduate nurses. *Journal of Advanced Nursing*. 1998;28(5):1134-45.

16. Maxfield D, Grenny J, Patterson K, McMillan R, Switzler A. *Silence Kills: The Seven Crucial Conversations for Healthcare*. Provo, UT: VitalSmarts; 2005. http://www.aacn.org/WD/Practice/Docs/PublicPolicy/SilenceKills.pdf.

17. Joint Commission. Behaviors that undermine a culture of safety. *Sentinel Event Alert*. 2008;40(9):1-5. https://www.jointcommission.org/assets/1/18/SEA_40 .PDF.

18. Bandura A. Moral disengagement in the perpetration of inhumanities. *Personality and Social Psychology Review*. 1999;3:193-209.

19. Neff K. Managing physicians with disruptive behavior. In Ransom SB, Pinsky WW, Tropman JE, eds. *Enhancing Physician Performance: Advanced Principles of Medical Management*. Tampa, FL: American College of Physician Executives; 2000:49-77.

20. Sotile WM, Sotile MO. The angry physician—part 2: Managing yourself while managing others. *Physician Executive*. 1996;22(9):39-42.

21. Sotile WM, Sotile MO. The angry physician—part 1: The temper-tantruming physician. *Physician Executive.* 1996;22(8):30-34.

22. Bernstein A. *Emotional Vampires: Dealing with People Who Drain You Dry.* New York: McGraw-Hill; 2001.

23. Buckman R. *How to Break Bad News.* Baltimore, MD: Johns Hopkins University Press; 1992.

24. Reason J. *Managing the Risks of Organizational Accidents.* Aldershot, UK: Ashgate; 1997.

25. Dwyer J. *Primum non tacere*: An ethics of speaking up. *Hastings Center Report.* 1994;24(1):13-18.

26. Kurkjian S. Stolen beauty: The Gardner Museum heist—15 years later. Secrets behind the largest art theft in history. *Boston Globe.* March 13, 2005. http://www.boston.com/news/specials/gardner_heist/heist/.

Chapter 5. Humility

1. Anderson PAM. Giving feedback on clinical skills: Are we starving our young? *Journal of Graduate Medical Education.* June 2012:154-58.

2. Coulehan J. "A gentle and humane temper": Humility in medicine. *Perspectives in Biology and Medicine.* 2011;54(2):206-16.

3. Epstein M. *Thoughts without a Thinker.* New York: Basic Books; 1995.

4. Gildas M. St. Bernard of Clairvaux. In *The Catholic Encyclopedia.* New York: Appleton; 1907. http://www.newadvent.org/cathen/02498d.htm. Accessed Feb. 26, 2017.

5. Bernard of Clairvaux. Sermon 42 on Canticle 6. In Burch GB, trans. *Introduction to Bernard's the Steps of Humility.* Cambridge, MA: Harvard University Press; 1942:51.

6. Meyer JR. St. Bernard de Clairvaux. *Encyclopaedia Britannica.* https://www.britannica.com/biography/Saint-Bernard-de-Clairvaux. Last updated Dec. 19, 2014.

7. Carota P. The word humble comes from Latin word "humus" earth from which God made us. *Traditional Catholic Priest.* http://www.traditionalcatholicpriest.com/2014/10/24/the-word-humble-comes-from-latin-word-humus-earth-from-which-god-made-us/. Published Oct. 24, 2014.

8. Richards N. Is humility a virtue? *American Philosophical Quarterly.* 1988;25(3):253-59.

9. Judge TA, Kammeyer-Mueller JD. On the value of aiming high: The causes and consequence of ambition. *Journal of Applied Psychology.* 2012;97(4):758-75.

10. Tangney JP. Humility. In Lopez S, Snyder CR, eds. *The Oxford Handbook of Positive Psychology.* 2nd ed. New York: Oxford University Press; 2009:483-90.

11. Tangney JP. Humility: Theoretical perspectives, empirical findings and directions for future research. *Journal of Social and Clinical Psychology.* 2000;19(1):70-82.

12. Leary MR, Bednarski R, Hammon D, Duncan T. Blowhards, snobs, and narcissists. In Kowalski R, ed. *Aversive Interpersonal Behaviors.* New York: Springer; 1997:111-31.

13. Miles RW. Fallacious reasoning and complexity as root causes of clinical inertia. *Journal of the American Medical Directors Association.* 2007;8(6):349-54.

14. Fowler J, Johnson D. On overconfidence. *Seed Magazine*. Jan. 7, 2011. http://seedmagazine.com/content/article/on_overconfidence/.

15. Peterson C, Seligman M. *Character Strengths and Virtues: A Handbook and Classification*. New York: Oxford University Press; 2004:461-75.

16. Johnson M, Patching GR. Self-esteem dynamics regulate the effects of feedback on ambition. *Individual Differences Research*. 2013;11(2):44-58.

17. Chatterjee A, Hambrick DC. It's all about me: Narcissistic chief officers and their effects on company strategy and performance. *Administrative Science Quarterly*. 2007;52(3):351386.

18. Ou AY, Tsui AS, Kinicki AJ, et al. Humble chief executive officers' connections to top management team integration and middle managers' responses. *Administrative Science Quarterly*. 2014;59(1):34-72.

19. Gabbard G. The role of compulsiveness in the normal physician. *JAMA*. 1985;254(20):2926-29.

20. Millon T, Davis RD. *Disorders of Personality*. 2nd ed. New York: Wiley; 1996:393-427.

21. Gunderson JG, Ronningstam E. Is narcissistic personality disorder a valid diagnosis? In Oldham JM, ed. *Personality Disorders: New Perspectives on Diagnostic Validity*. Washington, DC: American Psychiatric Press; 1991:107-19.

22. Kernberg O. Factors in the psychoanalytic therapy of narcissistic patients. *Journal of the American Psychiatric Association*. 1970;18:51-85.

23. Cooper A. Narcissism and masochism: The narcissistic-masochistic character. *Psychiatric Clinics of North America*. 1989;12(3):541-52.

24. Reason J. *Human Error*. Cambridge: Cambridge University Press; 1990:57-58.

25. Simon HA, Egidi M, Marris RL, Viale R. *Economics, Bounded Rationality and the Cognitive Revolution*. Brookfield, VT: Elgar; 1992.

26. Coulton GR. Hubris: The megaphone of overblown confidence. Linked 2 Leadership. https://linked2leadership.wordpress.com/2014/01/30/hubris-the-megaphone-of-overblown-confidence/. Published Jan. 30, 2014.

27. Croskerry P, Norman G. Overconfidence in clinical decision making. *American Journal of Medicine*. 2008;121(5A):S24-S29.

28. Meyer AN, Payne VL, Meeks DW, Rao R, Singh H. Physicians' diagnostic accuracy, confidence, and resource requests: A vignette study. *JAMA Internal Medicine*. 2013;173(21):1952-59.

29. Arkes H, Christensen C, Lai C, Blumer C. Two methods of reducing overconfidence. *Organizational Behavior and Human Decision Processes*. 1987;39:133-44.

30. Berner ES, Graber ML. Overconfidence as a cause of diagnostic error in medicine. *American Journal of Medicine*. 2008;121(5A):S2-S23.

31. Blanton H, Pelham BW, DeHart T, Carvallo M. Overconfidence as dissonance reduction. *Journal of Experimental Social Psychology*. 2001;37:373-85.

32. Croskerry P, Singhal G, Mamede S. Cognitive debiasing 1: Origins of bias and theory of debiasing. *BMJ Quality and Safety*. 2013;122:ii58-ii64.

33. Gandhi TK, Kachalia A, Thomas EJ, et al. Missed and delayed diagnoses

in the ambulatory setting: A study of closed malpractice claims. *Annals of Internal Medicine.* 2006;145(7):488-96.

34. Banja J. *Medical Errors and Medical Narcissism.* Sudbury, MA: Jones and Bartlett; 2005.

35. Johnson DDP, Blumstein DT, Fowler JH, Haselton MG. The evolution of error: Error management, cognitive constrains, and adaptive decision-making biases. *Trends in Ecology and Evolution.* 2013;28(8):474-81.

36. Christie W, Jones S. Lateral violence in nursing and the theory of the nurse as wounded healer. *Online Journal of Issues in Nursing.* 2014;19(1):1-10.

37. Critical Thinking Program. Dalhousie University website. https://medicine .dal.ca/departments/core-units/DME/critical-thinking.html. Accessed Oct. 6, 2018.

38. Maltsburger JT, Buie DH. Countertransference hate in the treatment of suicidal patients. *Archives of General Psychiatry.* 1974;30(5):625-33.

39. Armstrong A. What CS Lewis wrote is more powerful than what he didn't. *Blogging Theologically.* http://www.bloggingtheologically.com/2015/12/11/what-cs -lewis-wrote-is-better-than-what-he-didnt/. Published Dec. 11, 2015.

40. Owens BP, Johnson MD, Mitchell TR. Expressed humility in organizations: Implications for performance, teams, and leadership. *Organization Science.* 2013;24(5):1517-38.

41. National Academies of Sciences, Engineering, and Medicine; Institute of Medicine. *Improving Diagnosis in Health Care.* Balogh EP, Miller BT, Ball J, eds. Washington, DC: National Academies Press; 2015:4.13-4.24. https://www.nap.edu /catalog/21794/improving-diagnosis-in-health-care.

42. Croskerry P. Critical thinking and decision making: Avoiding the perils of thin-slicing. *Annals of Emergency Medicine.* 2006;48(6):720-22.

43. Croskerry P. The importance of cognitive errors in diagnosis and strategies to minimize them. *Academic Medicine.* 2003;78(8):775-80.

44. Haidt J. The emotional dog and its rational tail: A social intuitionist approach to moral judgment. *Psychological Review.* 2001;108(4):814-34.

45. Vera D, Rodriguez-Lopez R. Humility as a source of competitive advantage. *Organizational Dynamics.* 2004;33(4):393-408.

Chapter 6. Some Theoretical Aspects of Vigilance and Risk Acceptability

1. Golding D, Tuler S. Risk and risk assessment. In Jennings B, ed. *Encyclopedia of Bioethics.* 4th ed. Farmington Mills, MI: Macmillan Reference; 2014:2873-81.

2. Carroll RL, Hoppes M, Hagg-Rickert S, et al. Enterprise risk management: A framework for success. American Society for Healthcare Risk Management. http:// www.ashrm.org/resources/patient-safety-portal/pdfs/ERM-White-Paper-8-29-14 -FINAL.pdf. Published Aug. 29, 2014.

3. Reeves AR. Standard threats: How to violate basic human rights. *Social Theory and Practice.* 2015;41(3):403-34.

4. Rawls J. *A Theory of Justice.* Cambridge, MA: Belknap Press of Harvard University Press; 1971.

5. Alpha Ecological. Do you know how many bugs there are in your peanut

butter? http://www.alphaecological.com/blog/do-you-know-how-many-bugs-are
-in-your-peanut-butter/. Published Nov. 19, 2015.

6. Hingston S. What are the chances? *Boston*. March 2016. http://www.boston
magazine.com/health/article/2016/03/20/amy-reed-morcellation/.

7. Ong MBH. NEJM editors: There will be no clarification for disputed power
morcellation story. *Cancer Letter*. March 25, 2016. https://cancerletter.com/articles
/20160325_2/.

8. Grady D. Amy Reed, doctor who fought a risky medical procedure, dies at 44.
New York Times. May 24, 2017. https://www.nytimes.com/2017/05/24/us/amy-reed
-died-cancer-patient-who-fought-morcellation-procedure.html.

9. US Food and Drug Administration. Quantitative assessment of the prevalence of unsuspected uterine sarcoma in women undergoing treatment of uterine
fibroids: Summary and key findings. FDA.gov. http://www.fda.gov/downloads/
MedicalDevices/Safety/AlertsandNotices/UCM393589.pdf. Published April 17, 2014.

10. Seidman MA, Oduyebo T, Muto M, et al. Peritoneal dissemination
complicating morcellation of uterine mesenchymal neoplasm. *PLoS ONE*.
2012;7(11):e50058. http://journals.plos.org/plosone/article?id=10.1371/journal.
pone.0050058.

11. Susman E. Big concerns about inadvertent use of morcellation in previously
undiagnosed uterine leiomyosarcoma. *Oncology Times*. 2011;33(10):64, 66–67. http://
journals.lww.com/oncology-times/fulltext/2011/05250/Big_Concerns_about_inad
vertent_Use_of_Morcellation.15.aspx.

12. Levitz J, Kamp J. A medical device sidelined, but too late for one woman.
Wall Street Journal. Nov. 21, 2014. http://www.wsj.com/articles/a-medical-device
-is-sidelined-but-too-late-for-one-woman-1416600067.

13. Voelker R. New morcellation system does not eliminate cancer risk. *JAMA*.
2016;315(19):2057.

14. US Food and Drug Administration. FDA discourages use of laparoscopic
power morcellation for removal of uterus or uterine fibroids [press release]. FDA.
gov. April 17, 2014. http://www.fda.gov/NewsEvents/Newsroom/PressAnnounce
ments/ucm393689.htm.

15. US Food and Drug Administration. FDA warns against using laparoscopic
power morcellators to treat uterine fibroids [press release]. FDA.gov. Nov. 24, 2014.
http://www.fda.gov/NewsEvents/Newsroom/PressAnnouncements/ucm424435
.htm.

16. Rosenbaum L. N-of-1 policymaking—Tragedy, trade-offs, and the demise of
morcellation. *New England Journal of Medicine*. 2016;374:986–90.

17. Siedhoff MT, Wheeler SB, Rutstein SE, et al. Laparoscopic hysterectomy
with morcellation versus abdominal hysterectomy for presumed fibroids in pre-
menopausal women: A decision analysis. *American Journal of Obstetrics and Gynecology*. 2015;212(5):591.e1–591.e8.

18. Prasad V, Vandross A, Toomey C, et al. A decade of reversal: An analysis of
146 contradicted medical practices. *Mayo Clinic Proceedings*. 2013;88(8):790–98.

19. Sedwick J. The health care risk management professional. In Carroll R, ed.

Risk Management Handbook for Health Care Organizations. 4th ed. San Francisco: Jossey-Bass; 2004:119–56.

20. Joint Commission. Sentinel events. *Comprehensive Accreditation Manual for Hospitals.* Jan. 2013. https://www.jointcommission.org/assets/1/6/CAMH_2012 _Update2_24_SE.pdf.

21. Reason J. *The Human Contribution.* Burlington, VT: Ashgate; 2008.

22. Jonsen AR, Toulmin S. *The Abuse of Casuistry.* Berkeley: University of California Press; 1988.

Chapter 7. Fifty Shades of Error

1. Ayd MA. A remedy of errors. *Hopkins Medicine.* Spring–Summer 2004:20–25.

2. Ofri D. Why physicians hate to admit their errors, even to themselves. *Washington Post.* Aug. 3, 2010. http://www.washingtonpost.com/wp-dyn/content /article/2010/08/02/AR2010080203771.html.

3. Leape LL. Error in medicine. *JAMA.* 1994;272(23):1851–57.

4. Brook OR, O'Connell AM, Thornton E, et al. Quality initiatives: Anatomy and pathophysiology of errors occurring in clinical radiology practice. *Radiographics.* 2010;30(5):1401–10.

5. McConnell MP. Why are medical malpractice cases so difficult? (And so expensive?). *Personal Injury Legal News.* May 16, 2012. http://www.allenandallen.com /blog/why-are-medical-malpractice-cases-so-difficult-and-so-expensive.html.

6. Reason J. Safety in the operating theatre—part 2: Human error and organizational failure. *Quality and Safety in Health Care.* 2005;14(1):56–60.

7. Robbennolt J. Apologies and medical error. *Clinical Orthopedics and Related Research.* 2009;467(2):376–82.

8. Wei M. Doctors, apologies, and the law: An analysis and critique of apology laws. *Student Scholarship Papers.* Paper 30. http://digitalcommons.law.yale.edu/cgi /viewcontent.cgi?article=1030&context=student_papers. Published Aug. 8, 2006.

9. King JH. *The Law of Medical Malpractice: In a Nutshell.* Nutshell Series. St. Paul, MN: West; 1986.

10. Mockenhaupt M. 2011. The current understanding of Stevens-Johnson syndrome and toxic epidermal necrolysis: Epidemiology and risk factors. *Expert Review of Clinical Immunology.* 2011;7(6):803–15.

11. Oakley A. Stevens-Johnson syndrome/toxic epidermal necrolysis. Derm Net New Zealand. At http://www.dermnetnz.org/topics/stevens-johnson-syn drome-toxic-epidermal-necrolysis/. Last updated Jan. 2016.

12. Makary M, Daniel M. Medical error: The third leading cause of death in the U.S. *BMJ.* 2016;353:i2139–43.

13. James JT. A new, evidence-based estimate of patient harms associated with hospital care. *Journal of Patient Safety.* 2013;9:122–28.

14. Shojania KG, Dixon-Woods M. Estimating deaths due to medical error: The ongoing controversy and why it matters. *BMJ Quality and Safety.* 2017;26:423–28.

15. Pronovost PJ, Goeschel CA, Wachter RM. The wisdom and justice of not paying for "preventable complications." *JAMA.* 2008;299(18):2197–99.

16. Catchpole K. Who do we blame when it all goes wrong? *Quality and Safety in Health Care*. 2009;18:3-4.

17. Cook R; Cognitive Technologies Laboratory, University of Chicago. How complex systems fail. http://web.mit.edu/2.75/resources/random/How%20Complex%20Systems%20Fail.pdf. Updated as Revision D (00.04.21) in 2000.

18. Reason J. Safety in the operating theatre—part 2: Human error and organizational failure. *Quality and Safety in Health Care*. 2005;14(1):56-60.

19. Reason J. *The Human Contribution*. Burlington, VT: Ashgate; 2008.

20. Federico F. The five rights of medication administration. Institute for Healthcare Improvement. http://www.ihi.org/resources/Pages/Improvement Stories/FiveRightsofMedicationAdministration.aspx. Accessed Oct. 6, 2018.

21. Graber ML, Franklin N, Gordon R. Diagnostic error in internal medicine. *Archives of Internal Medicine*. 2005;165(13):1493-99.

22. Groopman JE. *How Doctors Think*. Boston: Houghton Mifflin; 2007.

23. King S, Pronovost P. Rekindling the central fire: Stories can change your life. Developed from a keynote presentation at the Patient Safety Congress; March 14, 2003; Washington, DC. https://www.patientsafetygroup.org/resources /news0403_print.cfm.

24. Kahneman D. *Thinking Fast and Slow*. New York: Farrar, Straus and Giroux; 2011.

25. Chassin MR, Becher EC. The wrong patient. *Annals of Internal Medicine*. 2002;136:826-33.

26. Lyu HG, Cooper MA, Mayer-Blackwell B, et al. Medical harm: Patient perceptions and follow-up actions [published online ahead of print 2014]. *Journal of Patient Safety*. 2017;13(4):199-201. http://www.wapatientsafety.org/wp-content /uploads/2014/12/Medical_Harm___Patient_Perceptions_and_Follow_up.99712.pdf.

27. Gazoni FM, Amato PE, Malik ZM, Durieux M. The impact of perioperative catastrophes on anesthesiologists: Results of a national survey. *Anesthesia and Analgesia*. 2012;114:596-603.

28. American Medical Association. *Code of Medical Ethics of the American Medical Association: Council on Ethical and Judicial Affairs, Current Opinions with Annotations*. Chicago: American Medical Association; 2010:8.12.

29. Banja J. Does medical error disclosure violate the medical malpractice insurance cooperation clause? In Henriksen K, Battles JB, Marks E, Lewin DI, eds. *Advances in Patient Safety: From Research to Implementation*. Rockville, MD: Agency for Healthcare Research and Quality and Department of Defense—Health Affairs; 2005:371-81. AHRQ Publication No. 05-0021-3. http://www.ahrq.gov/sites/default /files/wysiwyg/professionals/quality-patient-safety/patient-safety-resources /resources/advances-in-patient-safety/vol3/Banja.pdf.

30. Banja J. *Medical Errors and Medical Narcissism*. Sudbury, MA: Jones and Bartlett; 2005.

31. Oh RC, Reamy BV. The Socratic method and pimping: Optimizing the use of stress and fear in instruction. *AMA Journal of Ethics*. 2014;16(3):182-86.

32. LeDoux J. *The Emotional Brain*. New York: Simon and Schuster; 1998.

33. Pyszczynski T, Greenberg J, Solomon S, Arndt J, Schimel J. Why do people need self-esteem? A theoretical and empirical review. *Psychological Bulletin.* 2004;130(3):435-68.

34. Schulz K. *Being Wrong: Adventures in the Margin of Error.* New York: Ecco Press; 2010.

35. Croskerry P. Bias: A normal operating characteristic of the diagnosing brain. *Diagnosis.* 2014;1(1):23-27.

36. Johnson DDP, Blumstein DT, Fowler JH, Haselton MG. The evolution of error: Error management, cognitive constrains, and adaptive decision-making biases. *Trends in Ecology and Evolution.* 2013;28(8):474-81.

37. Cosmides L, Tooby J. Knowing thyself: The evolutionary psychology of moral reasoning and moral sentiments. In Freeman RE, Werhane P, eds. *Business, Science, and Ethics.* Ruffin Series no. 4. Charlottesville, VA: Society for Business Ethics; 2004:91-127. https://pdfs.semanticscholar.org/fe54/834c5e85f 941918deb3363d3be8d766a2e8b.pdf.

38. Gerstein M. *Flirting with Disaster: Why Accidents Are Rarely Accidental.* New York: Union Square Press; 2008.

39. Thompson E. *Waking, Dreaming, Being: Self and Consciousness in Neuroscience, Meditation, and Philosophy.* New York: Columbia University Press; 2015.

40. Cook R; Cognitive Technologies Laboratory, University of Chicago. How complex systems fail. http://web.mit.edu/2.75/resources/random/How%20Com plex%20Systems%20Fail.pdf. Updated as Revision D (00.04.21) in 2000.

41. Reason J. Human error: Models and management. *BMJ.* 2000;320(7237):768-70.

42. Green M. Nursing error and human nature. *Journal of Nursing Law.* 2004;9(4):37-44.

43. Reason J. *Human Error.* Cambridge: Cambridge University Press; 1990.

44. Waring J, Harrison S, McDonald R. A culture of safety or coping? Ritualistic behaviors in the operating theatre. *Journal of Health Services Research and Policy.* 2007;12(suppl 1):S1:3-S1:9.

45. Leape LL. Reporting of adverse events. *New England Journal of Medicine.* 2002;347(2):1633-38.

46. Nalder E. Despite law, medical errors likely go unreported. Hearst Newspapers. Seattlepi.com. Sept. 26, 2010. http://www.seattlepi.com/local/article/De spite-law-medical-errors-likely-go-unreported-889076.php.

47. Weissman JS, Annas CL, Epstein AM, et al. Error reporting and disclosure systems: Views from hospital leaders. *JAMA.* 2005;293(11):1359-66.

48. Benn J, Arnold G, Wei I, Riley C, Aleva F. Using quality indicators in anaesthesia: Feeding back data to improve care. *British Journal of Anaesthesia.* 2012;109(1):80-91.

49. Kaldjian LC, Jones EW, Wu BJ, et al. Reporting medical errors to improve patient safety: A survey of physicians in teaching hospitals. *Archives of Internal Medicine.* 2008;168(1):40-46.

50. National Academies of Sciences, Engineering, and Medicine; Institute of Medicine. *Improving Diagnosis in Health Care.* Balogh EP, Miller BT, Ball J, eds.

Washington, DC: National Academies Press; 2015. https://www.nap.edu/catalog
/21794/improving-diagnosis-in-health-care.

51. Schulman KA, Berlin JA, Harless W, et al. The effect of race and sex on physicians' recommendations for cardiac catheterization. *New England Journal of Medicine.* 1999;340(8):618-26.

52. Nouri SS, Rudd RE. Health literacy in the "oral exchange": An important element of patient-provider communication. *Patient Education and Counseling.* 2015;98(5):565-71.

53. Robert Wood Johnson Foundation. OpenNotes. https://www.rwjf.org/en/how -we-work/grants-explorer/featured-programs/opennotes.html. Accessed Oct. 6, 2018.

54. De Feijeter JM, de Grave WS, Muijtjens AM, Scherpbier AJJA, Koopmans RP. A comprehensive overview of medical error in hospitals using incident-reporting systems, patient complaints and chart review of inpatient deaths. *PLoS One.* 2012;7(2):e31125. http://journals.plos.org/plosone/article?id=10.1371 /journal.pone.0031125.

55. Croskerry P. Critical thinking and decision making: Avoiding the perils of thin-slicing. *Annals of Emergency Medicine.* 2006;48(6):720-22.

56. Graber M, Kissam S, Payne VL, et al. Cognitive interventions to reduce diagnostic error: A narrative review. *BMJ Quality and Safety.* 2012;21(7):535-57.

57. Van der Berge K, Mamede S. Cognitive diagnostic error in internal medicine. *European Journal of Internal Medicine.* 2013;24(6):525-29.

58. Mamede S, van Gog T, van der Berge K, et al. Effect of availability bias and reflective reasoning on diagnostic accuracy among internal medicine residents. *JAMA.* 2010;304(11):1198-1203.

59. Miles RW. Fallacious reasoning and complexity as root causes of clinical inertia. *Journal of the American Medical Directors Association.* 2007;8(6):349-54.

60. Amalberti R, Auroy Y, Berwick D, Barach P. 5 system barriers to achieving ultrasafe health care. *Annals of Internal Medicine.* 2005;142(9):756-64.

61. Redelmeier DA, Ferris LE, Tu JV, Hux JE, Schull MJ. Problems for clinical judgment: Introducing cognitive psychology as one more basic science. *Canadian Medical Association Journal.* 2001;164(3):358-60.

62. Berner ES, Graber ML. Overconfidence as a cause of diagnostic error in medicine. *American Journal of Medicine.* 2008;121(5A):S2-S23.

Chapter 8. The Standard of Care and Medical Malpractice
Law as Ethical Achievement

1. King JH. *The Law of Medical Malpractice: In a Nutshell.* Nutshell Series. St. Paul, MN: West; 1986.

2. Hall MA. The defensive effect of medical practice policies in malpractice litigation. *Law and Contemporary Problems.* 1991;54(2):119-45.

3. Gifis SH. *Barron's Law Dictionary.* Hauppauge, NY: Barron's Educational Series; 1984.

4. Dobbs DB, Keeton RE, Owen DG. *Prosser and Keeton on Torts.* 5th ed. St. Paul, MN: West; 1984.

5. Taylor C. The use of clinical practice guidelines in determining standard of care. *Journal of Legal Medicine*. 2014;35:273-90.

6. Bayles MD. *Professional Ethics*. 2nd ed. Belmont, CA: Wadsworth; 1989.

7. Mehlman MJ. Professional power and the standard of care in medicine. *Arizona State Law Journal*. 2012;44:1165-1235.

8. See, for example, Daubert v. Merrell Dow Pharmaceuticals, 590 US 579 (1993), which established a standard for admissibility of scientific testimony in US courts.

9. Huey K. Oct. 10, 2012. Medical necessity: What is it? Presentation for the American Academy of Professional Coders; Oct. 10, 2012; Chicago, IL. http://static.aapc.com/a3c7c3fe-6fa1-4d67-8534-a3c9c8315fao/cfa2b133-ce13-47e1-90c1-4907eba70dbd/6b9dc000-0897-4c24-9f4a-519e1f3ab372.pdf.

10. Rich BA. Medical custom and medical ethics: Rethinking the standard of care. *Cambridge Quarterly of Healthcare Ethics*. 2005;14:27-39.

11. Brownlee S. *Overtreated: Why Too Much Medicine Is Making Us Sicker and Poorer*. New York: Bloomsbury; 2007.

12. Mendelson TB, Meltzer M, Campbell EG, Caplan AL, Kirkpatrick JN. Conflicts of interest in cardiovascular clinical practice guidelines. *Archives of Internal Medicine*. 2011;171(6):577-84.

13. Livingston EH, McNutt RA. The hazards of evidence-based medicine: Assessing variations in care. *JAMA*. 2011;306(7):762-63.

14. Amdur RJ, Bankert EA. *Institutional Review Board: Member Handbook*. 2nd ed. Sudbury, MA: Jones and Bartlett; 2007.

15. Prasad V, Vandross A, Toomey C, et al. A decade of reversal: An analysis of 146 contradicted medical practices. *Mayo Clinic Proceedings*. 2013;88(8):790-98.

16. What conclusions has *Clinical Evidence* drawn about what works, what doesn't based on randomised controlled trial evidence? BMJ *Clinical Evidence* website. http://clinicalevidence.bmj.com/x/set/static/cms/efficacy-categorisations.html. Last updated Aug. 18, 2017.

17. Cahana A, Mauron A. The story of Vioxx—no pain and a lot of gain: Ethical concerns regarding conduct of the pharmaceutical industry. *Journal of Anesthesia*. 2006;20:348-51.

18. Solomon M. *Making Medical Knowledge*. Oxford: Oxford University Press; 2015.

19. Demetriades D, May A, Gamble H. When does a Centers for Disease Control and Prevention recommendation become standard of care? Perhaps in the courtroom. American College of Surgeons mock trial: Line sepsis liability. *Journal of the American College of Surgeons*. 2008;206(2):370-75.

20. Centers for Disease Control and Prevention. Guidelines for the prevention of intravascular catheter-related infections. *Morbidity and Mortality Weekly Report*. 2002;51(RR-10):1-36. https://www.cdc.gov/mmwr/pdf/rr/rr5110.pdf.

21. Adam Webb, MD, personal communication, Nov. 9, 2016.

22. Rizzo E. Top ten patient safety issues for 2014. *Becker's Infection Control and Clinical Quality*. Dec. 3, 2013. http://www.beckershospitalreview.com/quality/top-10-patient-safety-issues-for-2014.html.

23. Reason J. *The Human Contribution*. Burlington, VT: Ashgate; 2008.

24. Reason J. *Human Error*. Cambridge: Cambridge University Press; 1990:173–216.

25. Greenberg MD. Medical malpractice and new devices: Defining an elusive standard of care. *Health Matrix: Journal of Law Medicine*. 2009;19:423-45.

26. Hall MA. The defensive effect of medical practice policies in malpractice litigation. *Law and Contemporary Problems*. 1991;54(2):119-45.

27. Chesanow N. Malpractice: When to settle a suit and when to fight. *Medscape*. Sept. 25, 2013. http://www.medscape.com/viewarticle/811323_3.

28. McCannon J, Berwick DM. A new frontier in patient safety. *JAMA*. 2011;305(21):2221-22.

29. National Academies of Sciences, Engineering, and Medicine; Institute of Medicine. *Improving Diagnosis in Health Care*. Balogh EP, Miller BT, Ball J, eds. Washington, DC: National Academies Press; 2015. https://www.nap.edu/catalog/21794/improving-diagnosis-in-health-care.

30. Green M. Nursing error and human nature. *Journal of Nursing Law*. 2004;9(4):37-44.

31. Minkoff H, Ecker J. Genetic testing and breach of patient confidentiality: Law, ethics and pragmatics. *American Journal of Obstetrics and Gynecology*. 2008;198:498.e1-498.e4.

Chapter 9. The Present and the Future

1. Blanton H, Pelham BW, DeHart T, Carvallo M. Overconfidence as dissonance reduction. *Journal of Experimental Social Psychology*. 2001;37:373-85.

2. Fast facts—the nursing workforce 2014: Growth, salaries, education, demographics and trends. American Nurses Association. https://www.nursingworld.org/~4afac8/globalassets/practiceandpolicy/workforce/fastfacts_nsgjobgrowth-salaries_updated8-25-15.pdf. Updated Aug. 25, 2015.

3. Mukherjee S. The algorithm will see you now. *New Yorker*. April 3, 2017:46-53.

4. Hofmann BM. Too much technology. *BMJ*. 2015;350:h705. https://nhsreality.files.wordpress.com/2015/02/too-much-technology-hofmann.pdf.

Index